PATHS TO EXCELLENCE

Paths to Excellence

THE DELL MEDICAL SCHOOL AND
MEDICAL EDUCATION IN TEXAS

Kenneth I. Shine MD and Amy Shaw Thomas JD

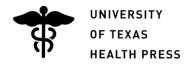

UNIVERSITY
OF TEXAS
HEALTH PRESS

Requests for permission to reproduce material from this work should be sent to:
    Permissions
    University of Texas Press
    P.O. Box 7819
    Austin, TX 78713–7819
    utpress.utexas.edu/rp-form

♾ The paper used in this book meets the minimum requirements of
ANSI/NISO Z39.48–1992 (R1997) (Permanence of Paper).

LIBRARY OF CONGRESS CATALOGING-IN-PUBLICATION DATA
Names: Shine, Kenneth I., author. | Shaw Thomas, Amy, author.
Title: Paths to excellence : the Dell Medical School and medical education in Texas /
    Kenneth I. Shine and Amy Shaw Thomas.
Description: First edition. | Austin : University of Texas Health Press, 2021. | Includes
    bibliographical references and index.
Identifiers: LCCN 2021008775 (print) | LCCN 2021008776 (ebook)
    ISBN 978-1-4773-2468-4 (hardcover)
    ISBN 978-1-4773-2469-1 (library ebook)
    ISBN 978-1-4773-2470-7 (non-library ebook)
Subjects: LCSH: Dell Medical School—History. | Dell Medical School—Finance. | Dell
    Medical School—Planning. | Educational fund raising—Texas—Austin. | Medical
    colleges—Texas.
Classification: LCC R747.D45 S55 2021 (print) | LCC R747.D45 (ebook) |
    DDC 610.71/176431—dc23
LC record available at https://lccn.loc.gov/2021008775
LC ebook record available at https://lccn.loc.gov/2021008776

doi: 10.7560/324684

CONTENTS

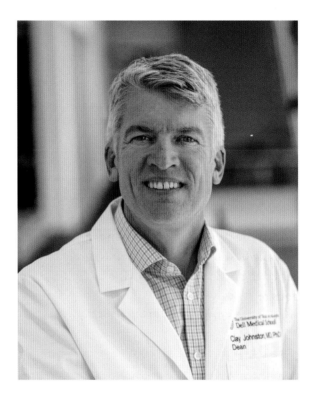

Clay Johnston

FOREWORD

When I first started telling people I was moving to Austin to help start a new medical school at the University of Texas, I was often met with quizzical looks. "Hasn't there *always* been a medical school there?" How could it be that the highly educated, progressive, and 11th largest city in the US and the flagship public university of the State of Texas did not have a medical school? The answer to this question is not simple, and it is certainly not dull, with twists and turns, steps forward, and disastrous retreats over decades.

Beginning with a fateful vote in 1881, the State of Texas split its first public medical school, sited in the population center of Galveston, from its flagship university in the capital city. That set in motion a structural division between health and academic campuses that would play out over a hundred years in the growing metropolitan areas of Texas. While seen as an impediment to research and education early on, most famously in Abraham Flexner's 1910 report on medical education, it remained the standard and a barrier to UT Austin simply starting its own medical school under its large umbrella of programs. Through the decades, many attempts were made to launch a medical school at UT Austin, all with popular support, political maneuvering, and a variety of financial plans, but each of these attempts failed.

Finally, a group of leaders came together in the early 2000s to piece together a solution, with key roles played by the UT System's Kenneth I. Shine, Executive Vice Chancellor of Health Affairs, and Amy Shaw Thomas, Vice Chancellor and Counsel for Health Affairs. As the architects of the solution and the authors of this book, their insights as insiders are particularly enlightening. There was a host of characters representing an array of civic and private entities, all with different interests. After several good attempts were stymied by natural and economic disasters, it all came together thanks to a resounding vote of support from the citizens of Travis County.

As the inaugural dean at Dell Medical School, I knew that much work had been done well before I arrived on the scene, with the foundations of the school and its mission already stably laid. However, I had no idea of the magnitude and complexity of the work, nor did I appreciate the potential value of learning about failed attempts before the final plan was set in motion. With this history, it is clear to me that those of us arriving after 2014 were simply carpenters building a structure that was designed for success by those who came before us. The mission of Dell Medical School is to revolutionize how people get and stay healthy, and its vision is a vital, inclusive health ecosystem. Ambitious and iconoclastic yet collaborative and community-oriented, these statements may have been written in the post-2014 era, but the concepts were established by those who came before, distilling the spirit of the people of the city and the university. Herein lies the complete story, as told by the two essential architects of a new, shining, audacious medical school at the University of Texas at Austin.

Clay Johnston, MD
Founding Dean, Dell Medical School

PREFACE

The establishment of a new allopathic medical school is a relatively uncommon event. The creation of a new medical school on an Association of American Universities campus during the past fifty years is particularly rare. The Dell Medical School resulted from a particularly interesting set of circumstances. The leadership of the University of Texas at Austin (UT Austin) campus did not initially favor a new medical school, which they saw as potentially draining resources such as state funding and philanthropy, from existing campus programs and priorities. The Texas Higher Education Coordinating Board had strongly urged that any new medical school in Texas be located in South or West Texas. State legislative funding of UT Austin had been declining for many years. Texas A&M University, fearful of the impact of a new medical school in Austin, established a satellite health campus in Round Rock, just north of Austin. Certain members of the University of Texas System Board of Regents (Regents) thought a new medical school at UT Austin would compete for resources with UT schools in their local communities and, in some cases, potentially outshine those institutions.

In spite of all of these obstacles, residents of Austin and many of its community organizations strongly supported the creation of a medical school in Austin. Many alumni and community leaders believed

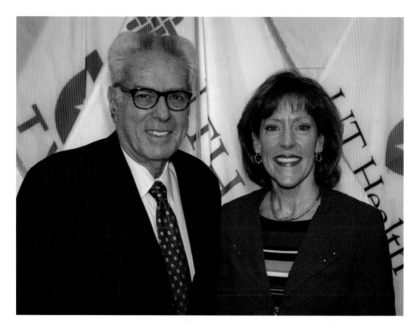

Kenneth Shine and Amy Shaw Thomas

that UT Austin would never be a truly great university without a medical school. Many faculty on the campus believed that their research would be significantly enhanced through collaboration with medical school faculty. Even Abraham Flexner, in his landmark 1910 study of American medical schools, argued for a medical school in Austin. The business community saw potential economic benefit from a local medical school, and some business leaders believed that a medical school would help recruit business executives and their families to Austin. A major health system in Austin, the Seton Healthcare Family (now Ascension Health), which had supported medical education for decades, recognized the advantage of medical research and recruiting local physicians, and recognized the other benefits that would result from a local medical school.

Over an eight-year period, a group of local leaders, UT System Board of Regents Chair James Huffines, and members of the UT System Office of Health Affairs aggressively developed and implemented plans to start a new medical school and expand the healthcare infrastructure in Austin and Central Texas. Gradually they convinced the Regents of the value of a new UT medical school in Austin. This was facilitated to some degree by the initiative for a new UT medical school in South Texas (the UTRGV School of Medicine), for which there was eventually broad Regental and legislative support when combined with a newly merged academic university in the Rio Grande Valley.

In Austin, a plan was developed to combine local hospital district tax monies with the residency training support of the Seton Healthcare Family to provide funding for a new medical school. Most importantly, a local state senator, Kirk Watson, provided brilliant leadership to advance and finance the school, along with many other aspects of his "10 in 10" proposals. After recovery from the severe economic recession of 2008, all this came to fruition, and the Regents approved the creation and financial support of a new medical school at UT Austin with the unique feature of local ad valorem tax support for operations of the school, with no new state monies.

This book is the story of these adventures. It starts with a discussion of how all the medical schools in Texas were created and exist separately from a general academic university campus and how the Dell Medical School became the first. (The UTRGV School of Medicine also became a part of the newly merged university in South Texas.) It tells the story of the prolonged efforts to start a medical school in Austin since the earliest days of the University of Texas. The book is based on the knowledge of the authors, who were active in the events, and is based on their interviews with many of the key participants. In the first few years, the Dell Medical School has already demonstrated its commitment to excellence, and its outstanding academic leadership has developed a unique national reputation in early fulfillment of many of the aspirations of the founders. We believe that years from now it will be counted as one of America's great institutions.

Kenneth I. Shine, MD
Amy Shaw Thomas, JD

ACKNOWLEDGMENTS

Many, many people contributed to the establishment of the Dell Medical School. A number of the key participants are identified in this book, yet the omission of others is a limitation of space and does not in any way lessen their efforts. Several individuals reviewed the text and made important contributions to the story. These include Charles Barnett, Kirk Watson, Sue Cox, and Steve Leslie, to whom we are very grateful. Trisha Meloncon, LuAnn Berger, and Lori Cook were especially helpful in facilitating its production. Special thanks to Robert Thomas for his strong support and good counsel. To all of these individuals we are very grateful.

PATHS TO EXCELLENCE

INTRODUCTION

In the spring of 2016, the first fifty medical students matriculated at the Dell Medical School, on the campus of the University of Texas at Austin (UT Austin). For over 131 years, this flagship academic campus lacked a medical school. Instead, the first medical school in the University of Texas was established by a vote of the people of Texas in 1881, as the UT Medical Department in Galveston. While the medical school in Galveston reported administratively to the President of the "main university," meaning UT Austin, it operated largely as a separate campus. This culminated in the establishment of a separate health science center in Galveston in 1967, which became the University of Texas Medical Branch at Galveston (UT Medical Branch, or UTMB). It was not until May 3, 2012, that the University of Texas System (UT System) Board of Regents voted to create a medical school in Austin. This book describes the long and often tortuous pathway to this accomplishment.

The precedent created by establishing a medical school geographically separate from the main academic campus in Austin was followed in the UT System by the establishment of medical schools in Dallas, San Antonio, and Houston, none of which were part of an academic campus. At the time the medical school in Austin was started, the UT System Board of Regents (Board of Regents) also established a new UT academic institution in South Texas by combining the University of

Texas–Pan American and the University of Texas–Brownsville into the University of Texas–Rio Grande Valley (UTRGV). This new university also included a new medical school. As a result, two academic campuses of the UT System included a medical school.

Although medical schools were established on the campuses of Texas A&M University (Texas A&M) and Texas Tech University (Texas Tech), a majority of their educational and research activities took place at distant locations. The Texas A&M medical school was administratively part of a separate health campus until the Texas A&M System merged it into the main academic campus in College Station in 2012. The only long-standing private medical school in Texas initially became part of Baylor University in 1903, although in a different city than the academic campus. Subsequently, even that medical school separated from Baylor and became the independent Baylor College of Medicine, in Houston.

Thus, medical schools and academic campuses were largely separate in Texas. For over a century, the UT System considered attempts to move the first UT medical school from Galveston to Austin and, subsequently, to create a new medical school on the flagship campus.

The separation of academic and medical campuses has had many consequences. Academic campuses are described as those that offer a broad range of course content and research, not including a medical school. They may include other professional schools such as a law school. Many faculty members on academic campuses work on projects in which there would be substantial advantages from a collaboration with physicians and other health professional faculty. This may involve applications of new technology, a device, or a potential drug, or new concepts in the prevention and treatment of disease. In the absence of a medical school, faculty members must often find collaborators at distant institutions to maximize complementary expertise and potential synergies. At times, grant applications fail, despite the fact that, had the medical school and academic faculties been on the same campus, the faculty of both institutions would have benefited from well-established collaborations.

Conversely, there is a valuable opportunity for medical school faculty to develop close interactions with faculty co-located on an academic campus. Both medical school faculty and academic faculty benefit from regular interactions in a number of disciplines. This includes not only the biological sciences, but also physical sciences and engineering, as well as opportunities to obtain doctoral degrees in disciplines ranging from economics to the behavioral sciences and master's degrees in a range of subjects, including business, e.g., the master of business administration degree. Dr. Abraham Flexner,[1] a renowned educator, pointed out the potential for these kinds of beneficial collaborations in his famous 1910 study of American medical schools on behalf of the Carnegie Foundation. Although UT Austin developed extremely well-funded research programs, if the campus had included a medical school the caliber of the University of Texas Southwestern Medical Center at Dallas (UT Southwestern), the combined research funding for UT Austin and UT Southwestern would have ranked UT Austin among America's top six research universities in 2010, resulting in higher national rankings and greater overall academic recognition for both institutions.

These arrangements did not mean, however, that separate UT System health science center campuses with medical schools did not have significant accomplishments. For over one hundred years, UT Medical Branch was the principal state institution caring for medically indigent patients who traveled across Texas to Galveston for their treatment. UT Medical Branch also became famous for its contributions to infectious disease, and the National Institutes of Health chose to build the highest-level infectious disease laboratory on the campus, one of only two such laboratories on academic campuses in the United States. UT Southwestern achieved international recognition for a broad range of contributions, especially related to cholesterol and cholesterol metabolism, for which Michael Brown and Joseph Goldstein received the campus's first Nobel Prizes. Ultimately, UT Southwestern employed as many as seven Nobel Prize winners. The University of Texas Health Science Center at San Antonio (UTHSC–San Antonio) conducts groundbreaking research in several areas, including geriatrics and diabetes, and has become a critically important healthcare institution for South Texas. The medical school at the University of Texas Health Science

Center at Houston (UTHSC-Houston) has a formidable clinical practice and became a central component of the Texas Medical Center, the largest medical center in the United States.

Although a member of the Association of American Universities (AAU), the nation's most distinguished institution for research universities, UT Austin was one of the very few AAU members without a medical school. Outside of Texas, only the University of California, San Francisco medical school achieved a top ranking in the United States without being an integral part of an academic campus.

For all these reasons and more, it was highly desirable for UT Austin to have a medical school. This finally came about because of a unique set of circumstances and opportunities.

The Texas Legislature historically showed little to no interest in supporting the funding and creation of a medical school in Austin. In 2002, the Texas Higher Education Coordinating Board (Coordinating Board) reported that any new medical school should be located in areas of underserved populations, including South and West Texas. The report did not support the establishment of a new medical school in Austin.

Like many of the previously created UT System medical schools, the local community in Austin became increasingly supportive of the need for a new medical school. Community organizations, particularly led by the Greater Austin Chamber of Commerce (Chamber of Commerce), argued that the city was becoming a major metropolitan area that would benefit substantially from biotechnology and health-related industries. In addition, there was a strong feeling by many business leaders, including Michael Dell, that a medical school in Austin would help recruit outstanding executives to their growing companies by assuring that they and their families would receive state-of-the-art care. While many individuals and organizations strongly supported a medical school, the critical need was for funding. It was clear that the state budget was tight and the Texas Legislature would not provide the funding. While many faculty at UT Austin wanted a medical school, campus leadership was concerned that a medical school would drain financial resources from the rest of the campus during a period of significantly decreased state funding for the university. Until a few years before the establishment of the new medical school in Austin, many members of the Board of Regents were also reluctant to see resources going to a new school at the expense of existing UT medical schools in their communities. However, many notable alumni of UT Austin believed that a medical school was an essential ingredient of a great university.

Key figures emerged who would influence and organize support for the new medical school. James Huffines was a prominent member of the Board of Regents from Austin who served two terms as Chair. He was a strong advocate for a medical school in Austin and worked to build support from other members of the board. State Senator Kirk Watson, from Austin, also played a pivotal role in the establishment of the new medical school, first in his capable overall support of the concept and, later, with his insightful development and advocacy of 10 Goals in 10 Years. These goals included building a medical school, a modern teaching hospital, and a cancer center, and improving mental health and ambulatory care in Austin, among others. Central to this activity was the concept that the newly established Travis County Healthcare District, which subsequently became known as Central Health, could use its property tax authority to support a medical school. Senator Watson had played a particularly important role in the creation of Central Health by virtue of carrying the bill in the Texas Legislature, which established the hospital district and authorized its taxing authority.

Ultimately, on May 3, 2012, the Board of Regents voted to provide substantial funding for the school if the local community would provide at least $35 million annually for the direct support of a medical school at UT Austin and if the Seton Family of Hospitals would continue to support residency training and clinical positions at current or increased levels. This was a unique concept. Although communities across the United States had voted for money to start a medical school, often these funds were earmarked for the land or construction of a hospital or other facilities, not a long-term commitment to support ongoing medical school operations.

Although the movement to start a new medical school in Austin was put on hold for several years because of the economic recession of 2007–2008, ultimately the voters of Travis County approved a Central Health property tax increase on November 6, 2012, that included the support of $35 million for the new medical school. The Board of Regents also allocated at least $25 million annually, with an additional $5 million per year for faculty recruitment for eight years. Susan and Michael Dell subsequently pledged $50 million to the new medical school in 2013, which was named in their honor and in recognition of a substantial amount of other funding they had previously provided to UT Austin. All new building construction related to the new medical school was funded through university debt.

Many community leaders played key roles in these developments, including Charles J. Barnett, FACHE, CEO of the Seton family of Hospitals; Greg Hartman, President and CEO of Seton Medical Center Austin (Seton) and Senior Vice President for Marketing, Communications and Planning; Rosie Mendoza and Clarke Heidrick, members of the Central Health Board; Trish Young Brown, CEO of Central Health; Michael W. Rollins, President of the Chamber of Commerce; Pete Winstead, founding partner of Winstead PC; and Joe Holt and Tim Crowley, banking executives. Additionally, from UT Austin and UT System, the following played an important role: Dr. Kenneth I. Shine, Executive Vice Chancellor for Health Affairs; Amy Shaw Thomas, JD, Vice Chancellor and Counsel for Health Affairs; Dr. Mark G. Yudof and Dr. Francisco Cigarroa, Chancellors; Dr. Randa Safady, Vice Chancellor for External Relations; and Dr. Steve W. Leslie, Provost at UT Austin.

Several issues emerge in understanding the development of the Dell Medical School at UT Austin. How did medical schools in Texas develop in a model that separated them from the main campuses of academic universities? What were the significant implications of this separation for the campuses and the medical schools? Why was it so difficult to create a medical school in Austin, and how were the obstacles to its founding overcome? How did UT Austin establish a medical school in Travis County without legislative approval and funding? The unique funding arrangements for the Dell Medical School required imagination, energy, creative solutions, and leadership in the face of resistance from the leadership at UT Austin. How did this evolve into a successful result? What are the short- and long-term prospects for the medical school? How did the development of a medical school in Austin impact the development of the school in South Texas, and vice versa? It is these questions this book attempts to answer. The authors believe that the unique origins of the medical school will help define its character in the future. The founding leadership of the school appears to support this idea.

CHAPTER 1

SEPARATION OF THE ACADEMIC UNIVERSITY AND MEDICAL SCHOOL

On September 15, 1883, classes began at the University of Texas[1] with 221 students (163 men, 58 women) and 8 male faculty. On April 21, 2014, almost 131 years later, ground was broken for the construction of the new Dell Medical School at UT Austin. By this point, the university had over 50,000 undergraduate and graduate students and more than 24,000 faculty and staff. Why had it taken so long for UT Austin to establish its medical school? How had this new medical school come about after all this time? What is the long-term significance of its establishment?

In 1929, UT Austin became a member of the prestigious Association of American Universities (AAU). The Dell Medical School was the first new medical school established on the campus of an AAU member in almost fifty years, and the majority of member universities already had medical schools. Outside of Texas, the principal AAU members without medical schools were institutes of technology such as Caltech, Georgia Tech, and Carnegie Mellon University. Notable exceptions were Princeton; the University of California, Berkeley; and the University of California, Santa Barbara.

Across the country, the vast majority of research-intensive medical schools were on academic campuses. Exceptions were the medical schools at the University of California, San Francisco, and all of the UT System medical schools. This separation also occurred in the Texas A&M and the University of North Texas systems. Furthermore, Texas Tech established the core of its medical school on its main campus in Lubbock but utilized regional campuses in El Paso, Amarillo, and Midland-Odessa. The Texas Tech campus in El Paso became a freestanding medical school and was named the Paul L. Foster School of Medicine in 2007, after Texas Tech received a $50 million gift from Foster, who also served on the Board of Regents of the UT System and as its Chair. In 2013, the Texas A&M System moved its medical school administratively into Texas A&M so that it would no longer be separate from the main university in College Station. Texas A&M continued to have sites at several locations, particularly in Temple, Texas. Developments to start a new medical school in Austin likely stimulated this change by the Texas A&M System. The only private medical school in the state, the Baylor College of Medicine, was originally part of Baylor University but became an independent institution in 1969. Another new medical school is developing as part of UTRGV, in South Texas.

As early as 1910, Dr. Abraham Flexner articulated the significant advantages of making a medical school part of an academic university. This was a major recommendation of his landmark report *Medical Education in the United States and Canada: A Report to the Carnegie Foundation for the Advancement of Teaching*, published that year. Yet this was not the case in Texas until recently.[2]

There are many benefits and synergies that arise when a medical school is part of a general academic university. Faculty in the medical school have opportunities to interact with other university faculty engaged in a broad diversity of activities, which may ultimately produce beneficial effects for the medical school. The relationship between engineering and medicine, including what has been called biomedical engineering, is just one example of these kinds of interactions. However, they exist in many other areas, such as the behavioral sciences, health economics, and other health professions, including nursing, pharmacy, and public health, as well as the natural and social sciences.

Co-location and integration on an academic campus allow health professional students to more easily obtain dual degrees, such as an MD with a master of business administration, or master of public health, or PhDs in a broad range of subjects, including the humanities and social sciences, as well as basic laboratory sciences.

EARLY DAYS OF MEDICAL SCHOOLS AND THE UNIVERSITY

In the earliest days, European medical schools were part of a larger university. These included institutions in London, Edinburgh, Paris, Bologna, and Vienna. From the eighteenth and nineteenth centuries into the early part of the twentieth century, many American physicians traveled to these European centers of excellence to further their education, if they could afford to do so. A number of these physicians returned to the United States, with very salutary effects on healthcare and medical education. In the United States, however, the relationship between the medical school and the university deserves attention when understanding the different evolution of medical schools in Texas.

In Colonial America and immediately thereafter, physicians were largely educated by apprenticeship to active practitioners. These apprentices would "shadow" the physician through practice and assist with treatments such as proper bandaging; applying leeches; bleeding; and dispensing a variety of medications, the most popular of which was chamomile. The period of apprenticeship was not fixed. Apprenticeships were extensively practiced in England, and America may have adopted that process from the English. The physician could then call himself "Doctor" (the overwhelming majority of physicians were men) and begin to practice. There were no examinations, no formal curriculum requirements, and no licensure. Most physicians were generalists, although beginning in the nineteenth century some began to specialize. As noted, physicians or students who could afford to do so traveled to Europe to learn their profession at a European university medical school. European medical training included extensive didactic instruction with lectures and demonstrations, with fewer practical clinical experiences during the educational process. However, the education was comprehensive, and the teachers were often experts in their fields.

William Shippen, the younger, returned to his native Philadelphia in 1762, after five years of study abroad, and began a series of lectures in midwifery and anatomy. His colleague John Morgan returned to Philadelphia shortly thereafter, and the two helped to found the school of medicine at the University of Pennsylvania, which is thought to be the first and only medical school in the original Thirteen American Colonies. This school established a precedent of being associated with and part of a university. The school of medicine added didactic lectures to the clinical experiences ordinarily found in apprenticeships. Shortly thereafter, a number of other universities, including Harvard, Yale, Columbia, and Dartmouth, established medical schools. Dr. Flexner noted that these additional medical schools were associated with their universities largely in name only, with neither financial support nor oversight from the university.

In the nineteenth century, there ensued an extraordinary proliferation of medical schools in the United States. Between 1810 and 1840, 26 new medical schools were established, and between 1840 and 1876, 47 more were created. Flexner reported that the number existing in 1876 had more than doubled prior to his study in 1910. Flexner observed that the United States and Canada had produced more than 447 medical schools in a little over a century. Many of these were short-lived, and Flexner indicated that at the time of his study there were 156 medical schools in the United States.

Flexner issued his groundbreaking report in 1910. During his study he visited all of the medical schools in the country, including "foreign" Texas. He concluded that of the four Texas medical schools, "there is only one medical school in the state fit to continue the work of training physicians."[3] This was the UT medical department at Galveston, Texas. Subsequently, Flexner states, "to the outsider it seems a regrettable mischance that located the medical department away from the university. Were it placed in Austin, it would apparently gain in every way: The town is as large and various state institutions there would strengthen its clinical opportunities; it would be easier to attract and to hold outsiders in teaching positions; the stimulus of the university would assist the growth of a productive spirit. . . . Perhaps it is not too late for the people of the state to concentrate their state institutions of higher learning in a single plant."[4] Therefore, Flexner recognized the inherent value of the co-location and integration of a medical school at the main University of Texas campus in Austin.

In his excellent history of American medical schools, Dr. William G. Rothstein points out that the majority of medical schools in the United States throughout the nineteenth and early twentieth centuries were proprietary schools.[5] Notable exceptions were the University of Pennsylvania and Johns Hopkins University. Proprietary schools had limited resources because they were owned by the faculty, and philanthropic support was very limited. Rothstein points out that in 1895 the Jefferson Medical College reorganized under a lay board of trustees "and put the faculty members on salary."[6]

The new leaders of medical education, particularly William H. Welsh at the Johns Hopkins University Medical School, argued that endowments would grow as philanthropists made donations to university medical schools. Research would prosper as medical school faculty members were appointed based on their research skills and adopted the values of university educators. The basic medical scientists would establish close ties with their counterparts in the university science departments, and laboratories would be used by both university and medical school students, thereby lowering costs. However, the Weiskotten Report, published in 1940 by Dr. Herman Weiskotten, Dean of the Syracuse University Medical School, demonstrated that "some schools of medicine have adopted a policy of complete isolation with reference to participation in the university's financial burdens, and have not readily undertaken additional responsibilities to fill the university's legitimate demands and have ignored all claims to attention on the part of the university."[7] Rothstein observed that the universities often diverted funds from the medical schools and used them for other purposes. He pointed out that the Weiskotten Report indicated "that the opinion was quite common that . . . medical schools had been governed best by being governed least."[8] Thus, it was only during the mid-twentieth century that firm and close relationships of medical schools with parent universities developed across the United States.

MEDICAL SCHOOLS IN TEXAS
BAYLOR

The challenges of building relationships between medical schools in Texas and parent universities are clearly exemplified by the history of the Baylor University College of Medicine, now the Baylor College of Medicine. The institution was created by a small group of Baylor University alumni physicians and opened October 30, 1900, as the University of Dallas Medical Department (even though there was no University of Dallas at the time). In 1903, the University of Dallas Medical Department aligned with Baylor University in Waco, and the name was changed to the Baylor University College of Medicine. It was one of four medical schools reviewed by Flexner in his 1910 report. Flexner was critical of the institution, arguing, "There is no clinical laboratory. Clinical opportunities are obtained at other institutions, but no infectious disease and little obstetrical work are obtainable. The clinical opportunities are thus decidedly inadequate."[9] Flexner reviewed two other Texas medical schools (the Fort Worth University Medical Department and the Southwestern University Medical College), both of which did not continue to function. By 1918, Baylor was the only private medical school in Texas. In 1943, when the MD Anderson Foundation invited Baylor to join the newly formed Texas Medical Center, in Houston, the school accepted the invitation. Under the leadership of preeminent surgeon Michael DeBakey, the Baylor University College of Medicine prospered. But in 1969, it separated from Baylor University and became an independent institution, named the Baylor College of Medicine, which is still the case today. There were multiple reasons for the separation, including "access to federal research funding" and a variety of governance issues. The Baylor College of Medicine remains the only private allopathic medical school in Texas.

THE UT HEALTH SCIENCE CENTERS
UT Medical Branch

An excellent history of the establishment of the UT Medical Branch is found in *The University of Texas Medical Branch at Galveston: A Seventy-Five Year History by the Faculty and Staff.*[10] The first university-based medical school in Texas was established in Galveston as the Medical Department of the Soule University on December 12, 1855, by the Texas Annual Conference of the Methodist Episcopal Church South. The governing board of the university created the chairs of law, medicine, and biblical science in 1857. Galveston was the logical place for the first university-based medical school since it was one of Texas's largest cities during this period and an active seaport. The Galveston Medical College, as the medical school became known, did not open until shortly after the end of the Civil War. A faculty of eight physicians began a series of lectures in November 1865. Twenty-three students entered the first class. Fees were advertised to be "$106.00 for the full course of lectures, $10.00 for tickets for dissections, a $5.00 onetime matriculation fee, and $20.00 for the diploma."[11] The graduation requirements included:

1. Three-year pupilage with a regular physician in good standing, inclusive of the time attending medical lectures in this college
2. At least one course of practical anatomy
3. Proper testimonials of character
4. An acceptable thesis in the handwriting of the candidate
5. A satisfactory examination in each of the departments of instruction
6. Candidates must be at least 21 years of age

Over several years, the faculty and the student body grew, but a series of "dissensions arose" involving Dr. Greensfield Dowell, the "leading spirit of the Galveston Medical College."[12] In 1873, the faculty resigned in a body, thus ending the first university-based medical school in Texas. A new school was created, the Texas Medical College and Hospital, over the next few years. Many of the students and some of the faculty of the Galveston Medical College joined the school. Dr. Ashbel Smith was the "driving force" behind it.[13] Smith is famous as a physician who graduated from Yale with bachelor and master of arts degrees in 1824 and an MD in 1828. He had a very distinguished career. As a close friend of Sam Houston, Smith was Surgeon General of the Republic of Texas Army in 1837. He was extraordinarily well educated, spoke several languages, and had "an accurate and extensive knowledge of Greek and Latin."[14] He was committed to patients in Texas and, because of his efforts, is often called the father of the University of Texas. Dr. Smith was a strong supporter of the Texas Medical College and Hospital, but when UT was established, he became a strong supporter of the first UT medical school.

In 1881, the Texas Legislature initiated plans to establish a university with a medical department and determined that the "people of Texas" would decide its location by popular vote. "At such locality as may be determined by a vote of the people, an institution of learning (shall be established) which shall be called and known as the University of Texas. The medical department of the university shall be located if so determined by a vote of the people, at a different point from the university proper, and as a branch thereof, and the question of the location of said department shall be submitted to the people and voted on separately from the proposition for the location of the main university. The nominations and locations for the medical department shall be subject to the other provisions of this act, with respect to the time and manner of determining the location of the university. The locality receiving the largest number of votes shall be declared selected and the university shall be established at such locale, provided that the vote cast for said locality shall amount to one-third of the votes cast."[15]

There were three parts to the ballot. The people of Texas could vote to place the entire University of Texas in a single city. The choices for this location included Austin, Waco, Albany, Graham, Williams Ranch, and Matagorda. Voters could choose to separate the main university from the medical department and place the main university in Austin, Lampasas, Caddo Grove, Peak, Thorps Springs, or Tyler, while placing the medical school in Galveston or Houston. Galvestonians felt that the medical school should be located in their city, particularly due to the presence of the Texas Medical College and Hospital, which were previously established in their community. The Texas Medical Association, during a meeting in Waco in April 1881, encouraged the selection of Galveston as the site for the new school. "The chief argument in favor of locating there was the fact that since Galveston was a seaport, it could supply a clinic with a variety of tropical and other diseases."[16] The vote was conducted on September 6, 1881. On October 17 of that year, the Texas Secretary of State, T. H. Bowman, revealed that the people of Texas had approved placing the medical department of the University of Texas apart from the main university in Austin. The vote in favor of a separate location was as follows: 38,117 for, 18,363 opposing. Galveston was chosen instead of its competitor, Houston, as the site of the University of Texas Medical Department by a vote of 29,741 to 12,586. Austin was chosen as the site of the main university.

Although the first session of the main university in Austin occurred on September 15, 1883, funding for the medical department in Galveston was not provided for five years, and the medical department did not begin until eight years after the main university opened. Of critical importance to the long-term future of the UT Medical Branch was the commitment of George Sealy and Rebecca Sealy to build the first John Sealy Hospital in Galveston in 1889, at a cost of $69,000. The hospital was named in honor of George Sealy's brother and Rebecca Sealy's late husband. John and Rebecca's children, John Sealy II and Jennie Sealy Smith, contributed to the long-term support and success of the UT Medical Branch by funding hospitals and healthcare on Galveston Island through the Sealy and Smith Foundation.

During this period, medical care in Texas was of very poor quality. "In 1891, 80% of the doctors in Texas had less than a year of formal medical training. It was an era of buffoonery and knavery. The cuppers and bleeders with some knowledge of herbs and dentistry ranked several degrees below cobblers in the estimation of the public. Diploma mills flourished."[17] The nation's death rate was triple that of today, and the average American's life span was forty-five years. The Roentgen X-ray had not been discovered, and yellow fever was an unchecked tropical menace.

In 1891, Regent Frank W. Ball moved at a Board of Regents meeting that "the medical department at Galveston be organized with the establishment of 8 distinct faculty with chairs, titles, and subjects to be defined at a later hour."[18] A faculty was recruited over the next several years, and the first faculty meeting was held on September 29, 1891. The formal opening of the medical school occurred on October 5, 1891. The first students were graduated in a relatively short time, on April 22, 1892. There were three graduates in 1892 and only one in 1893. A Dallas newspaper criticized wasting money on maintaining a medical school in Galveston with so few graduates. However, over the next several years the number of students and faculty gradually increased.

Marie Delalondre Dietzel was the first woman graduate of the medical school in 1897. The school continued to have financial difficulties, with major challenges meeting its payroll and functioning with limited resources. However, it did benefit dramatically by the construction, beginning in 1890, of a very large red-brick building, which became known as "Old Red." This building provided laboratory instructional space, including anatomy dissection rooms, for the school during its earliest years. It was one of the few buildings to survive the 1900 hurricane in Galveston. Old Red currently stands at UT Medical Branch as the Ashbel Smith Building.

During its earliest years, the medical department of the University of Texas at Galveston was viewed by many as an afterthought. The Texas Legislature was not particularly supportive of legislative funding, and the Board of Regents was not financially committed to the medical school. In 1893, a school of pharmacy was established as part of UT Galveston. It was the first school of pharmacy in Texas, and it subsequently moved to UT Austin in 1927.

Paradoxically, the hurricane of 1900 devastated Galveston but stimulated significant support from the Board of Regents for the medical school. Few structures survived the storm. Although damaged, Old Red was one of the few buildings that remained. In the aftermath of the storm came a telegram message that has become legendary. Beauregard Bryan, the Chair of the UT System Board of Regents Medical Committee, sent the message: "The University of Texas stops for no storm."[19] Both Regental and legislative financial support increased in the aftermath of the storm. In many ways, this was attributed to the resilience of the faculty, staff, and students at the medical school, who behaved responsibly during and after the storm and worked vigorously for the recovery of the school. In his commencement address in 1925, Dr. James E. Thompson, a professor of surgery, said, "Looking back it appears to me that this critical period was the turning point of our history. It was the first time that the Board of Regents dipped deliberately into the Available University Fund (AUF) to supply the needs of the medical department and this very act made us feel that our school really belonged to the current university and was not merely a stepchild. Further, the Board of Regents was so generous in repairing the damage to the buildings and restoring the equipment, they were actually in better shape at the end of the year 1901 than we had been before."[20]

The laboratories and equipment were upgraded with UT Regental support. This support was in significant contrast to that available after Hurricane Ike hit Galveston Island in 2008. In 1900, the medical department was part of the University of Texas and therefore eligible for AUF from the UT endowment. In 2008 the UT Medical Branch was a separate university and not eligible for AUF, which was available to fund operations only at UT Austin, the UT System Administration, and the Texas A&M System. Moreover, in 2008, the use of UT endowment monies for reconstruction was further limited, to maximize the amount of Federal Emergency Management Administration (FEMA) funding. The use of Permanent University Fund (PUF) monies for reconstruction prior to FEMA's support would have jeopardized the use of federal funds. Employee layoffs at UTMB and the limitations on funding caused renewed speculation about moving the medical school to Austin and, indeed, moving the whole campus. Nothing came of this speculation.

UT Austin was the original academic campus and considered its flagship. When the University of Texas created a medical school in Galveston, the individual responsible for that medical school reported to the President of the "main university," which was the term given for the role of the President at the University of Texas campus in Austin. Subsequently, multiple schools were developed at a variety of sites, all of which reported administratively to the President of the main university. In 1950, the Board of Regents concluded that there needed to be some identification of the various schools as part of a UT System and that the reporting relationships needed to be to the System, as opposed to the "president of the main university." On April 28, 1950, a chancellor was identified for the UT System as its chief administrative officer. Initially, the chancellor was the same individual who served as President of the UT Austin campus, but eventually it was determined that the individual who served as chancellor ought to be a different person than the President of UT Austin.

In summary, the 1881 political competition for the establishment and placement of UT resulted in the vote to allow the medical department and the main university to be located at different sites, which set the precedent in Texas for a medical school to be separate from the main academic university. Until 1967, the UT Medical Department was considered part of the main university in Austin, and the ultimate responsibility for the school was held by the President of the university. However, throughout that period the medical department was largely autonomous. Only when there was trouble in Galveston did the President of the main university in Austin get involved, as in the 1940s. But this was an infrequent event. Certainly, there were essentially no programs or academic activities that were conducted in close relationship to the Austin campus—a fact Flexner lamented as early as 1910.

Organizational diagrams through the years showed multiple health institutions reporting to the President of the main university in Austin. It was only after the establishment of a permanent Chancellor for the UT System in 1960 that a Vice Chancellor for Health Affairs, later known as the Executive Vice Chancellor for Health Affairs, provided the reporting line and oversight for the medical school. At the same time, the medical school could function quite independently of the main university in Austin. A number of attempts were made to move UTMB back to Austin, but all of these ultimately failed. The first President of the UT Medical Branch, Truman Blocker, was appointed in 1967, although he continued for a short time, at least on paper, to have a reporting relationship to the President of UT Austin.

UT Southwestern

A spring 2014 publication by the Southwestern Medical Foundation entitled *Southwestern Medical Perspectives* (*Perspectives*) provides an excellent history of the development of the next UT medical school, UT Southwestern, which occurred after a number of earlier failed attempts to create a permanent medical school in Dallas. The *Perspectives* history states, "While qualified and notable doctors were practicing medicine in Dallas at the time, many more were poorly trained, most received only basic training from small medical schools which required only one to two years of study following three years of high school. Fake medical licenses were common. An MD degree could be conferred by return postage in exchange for a letter of intent and a fee of $15.00. In fact, a stranger could come to town, say he was a doctor, register with the health officer, and be allowed to practice medicine."[21] As previously mentioned, the first attempt to start a medical school in Dallas resulted in the creation of the University of Dallas Medical Department, which became the Baylor University College of Medicine in 1903. In 1908, another attempt was made to create a medical school in Dallas under the name "Southwestern University Medical College." This institution received a negative assessment by Flexner and did not survive.

In the late 1930s, community efforts to create a medical school in

Dallas were once again energized, primarily by the philanthropic community. Dr. Edward H. Cary was a successful physician and businessman who saw the value of having an outstanding medical school in Dallas. In 1938, the Baylor University College of Medicine was in dire financial straits, conducting little research, and providing instruction primarily in the form of lectures. Cary dreamed of "a truly great Southwestern medical center," which he knew could develop only from sustained philanthropic and financial support. He combined forces with Karl Hoblitzelle, a philanthropist businessman, in an effort to create a medical school. They formed the Southwestern Medical Foundation on January 31, 1939, and both made major financial contributions to the foundation. "On March 8, 1942, Cary publicly communicated his vision for a strong medical center that would be spread across a 35-acre tract of land on Harry Hines Boulevard. The centerpiece of this vision, a new medical school, would be called Southwestern Medical College."[22] Baylor University College of Medicine was offered an opportunity to play a role in the development of this new medical center; however, shortly thereafter, Baylor accepted an offer from the MD Anderson Foundation to become part of the newly created Texas Medical Center, in Houston.

In spite of World War II, sufficient funds were raised to establish the Southwestern Medical College. Since major new construction was unfeasible during the war, a series of prefabricated plywood barracks were used to house the institution, which was accredited on December 15, 1943. Despite substantial progress in recruiting faculty and developing programs, the medical school lacked the additional resources needed to further develop and remain consistent with the founder's vision. In May 1949, the Texas Legislature passed a bill that allowed the creation of a new state medical school on the recommendation of the House of Delegates of the Texas Medical Association. The Southwestern Medical Foundation launched a major campaign on behalf of the medical school, identifying the faculty, student body, laboratories, research, and $1.5 million in assets held by the foundation that would become part of the medical school. The Texas Medical Association's House of Delegates voted 79 to 54 in favor of Dallas as the site of the new medical school. The Board of Regents unanimously accepted the transfer of assets and restricted funds on September 18, 1949, and, as a result, assumed the operations of the Southwestern Medical School of the University of Texas. The institution continued to thrive under outstanding leadership and has become one of America's great medical schools and health science centers.

UT Southwestern was not the result of any overall state plan for medical education but, rather, the result of efforts of local physicians and philanthropists who created an institution that was later transferred to UT. Therefore, a second medical school was established in the UT System apart from a general academic university, and it eventually became part of a health science center. There was no UT academic campus in Dallas at that time. UT Southwestern continues to benefit from a tradition of very strong community and philanthropic support. Some of its philanthropic supporters later expressed great concerns about the UT System establishing a medical school in Austin (during the planning for the new medical school) because it might create a serious competitor to their institution.

UTHSC–San Antonio

In the aftermath of WWII, returning veterans and the baby boom created a great need for more physicians in Texas. This desire was supported by additional federal funding for the expansion of medical school class sizes and the creation of new medical schools across the country. The number of four-year medical schools in the United States had fallen to 72 in 1949, possibly as a result of the Flexner Report. That number rose to 126 by 1983, for an increase of well over 50 percent. The majority of these new schools were public medical schools, which increased from 32 to 76, more than a twofold increase. Private medical schools increased from 40 to 50 during this time. The University of Texas Medical School at San Antonio was established, in large part, as a response to this need for more physicians.

Will C. Sansom, author of *The Crown Jewel: The Story of the First 50 Years of the University of Texas Health Science Center at San Anto-*

nio, has provided an excellent overview of the circumstances leading to the creation of the UT Medical School at San Antonio. The San Antonio area became a rapidly growing city and region of Texas, but it did not approach the number of physicians per person in Dallas and Houston. A Texas Medical Association survey of 6,000 physicians statewide "showed medical doctors were not evenly distributed across urban and rural areas, and that South Texas was in dire need of more physicians."[23] Studies also showed that "Texas was importing half of its licensed physicians from out of state."[24] In an argument that was later used in Austin, it was said that "the 1950 census showed San Antonio was one of the largest cities in the country not to have a medical school."[25] In the 1940s and 1950s, many community leaders and physicians worked to support a medical school in San Antonio. Sansom gives special credit to John M. Smith Jr., MD, Mirchen M. Mintor, MD, and James P. Holleis, DDS, as key community leaders who galvanized support for the medical school. At the same time, San Antonio was developing a variety of hospitals, including Brooke Army Medical Center (established in 1938) and Wilford Hall Medical Center (established in 1937), that made military healthcare training and medicine particularly important in the community.

In 1947, community leaders established the San Antonio Medical Foundation to "concentrate efforts on attaining a medical, dental, and nursing education center for the city and region."[26] Initially, the foundation acquired 200 acres for this purpose, which increased to 500 acres in the 1960s and has reached 900 acres today. The Medical Foundation offered land for the medical school and adjacent hospitals. In 1959, the Texas Legislature established the South Texas Medical School in San Antonio. The bill required that a suitable teaching hospital be constructed within one mile of the medical school. Subsequently, in January 1961, Bexar County voters overwhelmingly approved $5 million in bonds to build a teaching hospital, and $1.5 million to renovate the existing county hospital, the Robert B. Green Hospital, in downtown San Antonio. In February 1961, the Board of Regents authorized the creation of the South Texas Medical School. There would be another vote of registered voters six years later, to increase hospital district taxes. That ballot proposal, which required planners to increase their projections of the hospital's operating costs, would be defeated, setting the stage for a "trio of county commissioners to make a gutsy overrule of their own constituents."[27] Throughout this period, Austin was competing for a new medical school, without success.

Sansom comments, "Without question, positive economic backdrop, the community leaders' moxie, the military medical presence, the increasing need for physicians in South Texas, the growth of the city, the existence of a medical foundation, the availability of acreage, and the previous requests before the Texas Legislature were all factors that set the stage for a San Antonio medical school that later became a comprehensive health science center."[28]

A number of years passed before the first students matriculated at the San Antonio medical school. Fifteen students enrolled in September 1966 and were assigned to the University of Texas medical schools at Dallas and Galveston. In 1967, seven students were similarly enrolled at Dallas and Galveston. Fifty-six students began classes at the new facility at the San Antonio medical school in September 1968, at which time the second- and third-year students returned to San Antonio for the continuation of their studies.

On June 5, 1969, the Texas Legislature created the University of Texas at San Antonio as a general academic university. The donation of 600 acres in northwest San Antonio for the site of the new university resulted in a geographic separation between the newly created academic campus and the medical center site. Subsequently, a number of collaborative projects would develop between the two institutions, but they remained separate institutions.

Two studies were done to determine whether to merge UT San Antonio and UTHSC–San Antonio. In 2002, consultant Dr. Carol Aschenbrener conducted the first study, and in 2010, Dr. Peter Flawn led a special advisory group to the Board of Regents to examine a possible merger of the two institutions. Both case studies recommended against a merger, citing the different stages of development of the two UT campuses, the costs and complexities of a merger, and the opportunity for further collaborative initiatives that could be accomplished without a formal consolidation.

Again, the creation of a medical school in the UT System was driven by community leadership, energy, resources, and political acumen. As in Dallas, and later in Houston, a medical school was established in a community that did not have an academic university campus. During this period there were community efforts to start a medical school in Austin, but they were not comparable to the efforts in San Antonio. Moreover, the political leadership in San Antonio made a more effective case with the Texas Legislature.

UTHSC-Houston

The medical school at the UT Health Science Center at Houston (UTHSC-Houston) began in a very different manner than the preceding schools. It started as part of a series of health science schools coming together in Houston. The University of Texas School of Dentistry was initially founded in 1905 as a privately owned dental college. It joined UT in 1943 and reported to the main university in Austin. In 1941, MD Anderson Hospital was established in Houston. Two decades later, in 1962, the President of the hospital, R. Lee Clark, MD, led a movement to establish a graduate school of biomedical sciences in Houston. The graduate school was established on July 11, 1963, and became part of the UT System on September 28, 1963. The Hill-Burton Act of 1946 was then used to start and fund a school of public health. Although these funds were authorized for the UT School of Public Health in 1947, they were not provided until 1967, and its first class matriculated in 1969. A new UT school of nursing matriculated its first students in 1972.

The initiatives to increase the number of physicians throughout the state and country led the Texas Legislature to establish a medical school in Houston in June 1969. Its first class of nineteen students matriculated in 1970. In 1968, the Board of Regents had signed an affiliation agreement with the Hermann Hospital Estate to provide the principal teaching facility for the proposed school. This was an unusual example of a local hospital being directly affiliated with the Board of Regents rather than with the local medical school. In the absence of any buildings dedicated to the medical school, the first medical students were enrolled at other UT medical school campuses until June 1971, when a class of thirty-two students began their full four years in Houston. During this period, the Board of Regents believed that the city could support a medical school because of its size and wealth.

In 1972, all of these health professions schools, including the medical school, became part of UTHSC-Houston. In November 2015, in response to a substantial gift from the McGovern Foundation, the medical school was named the John P. and Kathrine G. McGovern Medical School. At the time of its creation, the UT medical school in Houston became part of the Texas Medical Center. Although another University of Texas institution, MD Anderson Cancer Center, was located in the Texas Medical Center, there was no academic University of Texas campus in Houston, which remains the case today. The medical school in Houston joined UT Medical Branch, UT Southwestern, and UTHSC–San Antonio as part of a health science center campus but not a general academic university campus.

THE EVOLUTION OF THE UNIVERSITY OF TEXAS SYSTEM

The UT System was established as a formal institution in 1950. At a meeting on April 28, 1950, the Chancellor of the UT System was identified as an officer of UT Austin. Other officers of the UT System included a Vice President of the UT Medical Branch. The presumption was that this individual would report to the President of the UT System's main university in Austin; however, during the early days of the UT System, the Chancellor and the President of UT Austin were often the same individual.

In 1967, the UT System created a full-time chancellor who was responsible for all of its campuses. Previously, chancellors had also been presidents of UT Austin. The Vice Chancellor for Health Affairs was responsible for UTMB; UT Southwestern; UTHSC–San Antonio; the dental branch in Houston; MD Anderson Cancer Center; continuing education in Houston; the public health school in Houston; and nursing schools in Austin, El Paso, Galveston, and San Antonio. Each of these entities had a Dean or Director, except for UT Medical Branch, which had a recently appointed President, as previously noted. All of the Houston schools (dentistry, nursing, public health, and the graduate school of biomedical sciences) were then combined with the medical school to create UTHSC-Houston. Two other medical schools were also incorporated into health science campuses, e.g., UT Southwestern and UTHSC–San Antonio. UTMB became a health science center with multiple professional schools, but the UTMB appellation persisted. The new medical schools in Austin and South Texas became part of the UT System by virtue of their creation within an overall academic campus.

CHAPTER 2

THE AUSTIN SCENE

Even though Texas voters in 1881 placed the first UT medical school in Galveston rather than in Austin, the citizens of Austin had not given up on having a medical school. Very little happened during the first half of the twentieth century with regard to additional UT medical schools in Texas. In 1941 the medical school did occupy the Regents briefly.[1] However, the 1940s saw the movement of the Baylor University College of Medicine from Dallas to Houston and the creation of a medical school in Dallas that would eventually lead to the second medical school in the UT System. In the early 1940s, the President of UT Austin was Homer Price Rainey. The Dean of the UT Medical Branch, in Galveston, was Dr. John W. Spies. President Rainey began to consider moving the medical school back to Austin. In 1942, there were faculty controversies at UTMB, which prompted legislators to also consider moving the school from Galveston to Austin. It was recognized that moving the medical school out of Galveston would require a constitutional amendment, and the "constant bickering" at UTMB led to state representatives being urged to do something about the situation.[2]

Shortly thereafter, the Medical Committee of the Board of Regents considered Rainey's recommendation to move the medical school to Austin. He argued that the schools (i.e., the academic campus and medical school) should "be concentrated here for the purpose of more cohesive training at a place that can provide adequate clinical materials."[3] The Sealy and Smith Foundation in Galveston pledged $2 million toward the construction of a new teaching hospital, which likely influenced the Regents' deliberations. The Regents' medical committee recommended that the medical school at Galveston be maintained there "permanently." By a vote of six to one on September 29, 1944, the Board of Regents accepted this recommendation. President Rainey was most disturbed by this action and said, "I feel we are making the most serious mistake that has ever been made."[4] However, Rainey had been embroiled in an intense controversy with the Board of Regents over issues of academic freedom and the political perspectives of some of the faculty members at UT Austin. Rainey, who vigorously defended both, was fired in November 1944, shortly after the Regents decided to adopt the medical committee's recommendation to keep the medical school in Galveston.

As previously noted, during the post–World War II era, there were national efforts to create new medical schools, and many people in Austin were anxious to have a school. Legislators introduced a number of bills during the 1949 Texas Legislature to create a second University of Texas medical school in Central Texas. San Antonio, Austin, Waco, and Temple were considered possible locations. By the mid-1950s, Austin community leaders and media were arguing that the city was well prepared for a medical school. On December 9 the advantages of an Austin medical school were summarized. These included four hospitals, a completely new and beautiful St. David's Hospital, the Austin State Hospital, a Cerebral Palsy Center, many state agencies, health departments and laboratories, and the location of the *Texas State Journal of Medicine* as among the reasons Austin would be recognized as the "medical center of Texas."[5] However, over the next four years, San Antonio's commitment of resources, including substantial amounts of land and its effectiveness in the political arena, resulted in its selection for the next UT medical school. An important factor in the decision was the rejection of Austin as a site by the Texas Medical Association at its annual meeting in Houston. The year before, the association had passed a resolution favoring San Antonio as the site of the next Texas medical school. A survey team from the Council on Medical Education of the American Medical Association (AMA) also supported San Antonio as the location of the school.

The City of Austin requested a similar study of Austin's suitability for a medical school, which was completed by the AMA in August 1958. The study recommended placing a new medical school adjacent to Brackenridge Hospital and emphasized the value of being in the same city as UT Austin, along with the importance of a close parent-university relationship. It also identified the libraries of UT Austin and the State Medical Association as important assets. Some citizens also preferred locating a new medical school on state land at the Austin State Hospital, or on the Austin "Hancock tract."

In the aftermath of the 1961 loss of the medical school to San Antonio, local physicians and citizens in Austin continued to argue for a medical school. They emphasized the concept of a basic science school focusing on the first two years of medical school. There were other sites for basic science medical schools in consideration, including Lubbock and Amarillo. The AMA's Council on Medical Education recommended that basic science schools be under the wing of strong major universities, which made the Austin location particularly attractive.

For several years thereafter, community groups in Austin continued to support either a two- or four-year UT medical school in Austin.[6] A 1961 study by faculty at the UT Medical Branch had proposed that a "crash program be adopted to set up a two-year basic sciences medical school at the main university."[7] Leaders in this effort argued that Austin was prepared to provide a site for such a medical school. The recommendations, written by Dr. Edwin G. Troutman, emphasized the importance of a medical school being a part of the main university. The report quoted Flexner, saying that he had "pleaded mightily for the incorporation of medical schools into the fold of the university, not just in name, but in toto, so that the medical faculty, curriculum, and students would be as much a part of the university as the other teachers and students, thereby preserving the requested scholarly atmosphere, for it is difficult to be inflamed with the study of learning elsewhere."[8] Troutman, of the Galveston medical faculty, was a frequent spokesperson, arguing, "Therefore it seems quite likely that a two-year basic sciences medical school in Austin would attract students of high quality and provide an impetus to the development of the science of medicine in Texas, as lending a more immediate partial remedy to the problem of physician supply in Texas."[9]

In 1967, in conjunction with the expansion of the Brackenridge Hospital and led by its President, William D. Youngblood, the Community Council of Austin and Travis County called for a new study on the possibility of a two-year medical school in Austin. Youngblood noted that voters had approved a $3.5 million bond issue for the Brackenridge expansion. The proposed study committee would update a 1964 recommendation and be charged with identifying the need for additional physicians in Texas, the effect of a medical school on the community and health services, and the economic value of a medical school. A number of community groups were invited to participate in the process. However, it is not clear that such a study was conducted at that time.

The Austin efforts suffered a serious setback in March 1967, when Frank C. Erwin Jr., the Chair of the Board of Regents, publicly said, "Austin is not prepared and will not be prepared in the near future for a traditional medical school." At a meeting with the Community Council of Central Texas Comprehensive Health Planning Commission, Erwin stated that Austin "cannot compete with Dallas or Houston for a University of Texas Medical School." He argued that a four-year medical school would require a teaching hospital with 800 to 1,000 beds and a closed medical staff. He estimated that a hospital that met such standards would cost the city more than $6 million per year. Meeting participants noted that this would involve a sizable local tax increase. Erwin argued that the cost of a medical student, at $15,000 per year, was "the most expensive of any educational area." He further argued that state funds were inadequate for UT to operate a medical school of high standards. Erwin said, "Austin is in no position to raise that money; it takes a metropolitan area such as Houston or Dallas, where their generosity has been proven to raise adequate supplementary, private, and foundation funds." He further commented, "Austin might leap the teaching hospital hurdle with a two-year medical school, but what faculty can be recruited to a two-year school? A two-year school cannot be staffed."[10] There was additional discussion about enhanced funding of patient care through the newly developed federal Medicaid program, and speculation that income from that program might help in the long-term support of a teaching hospital. At the same meeting, UT System Health Affairs Vice Chancellor Charles LeMaistre, MD, affirmed Erwin's warnings and argued that a two- or three-year medical school would become a "white elephant" in five or more years if it was not expanded to a four-year curriculum. Representatives of the Travis County Medical Society continued their support of a medical school and cited a report by Booz Allen Hamilton that recommended the creation of a medical school in conjunction with the Brackenridge Hospital, which the City of Austin was to enlarge to 500 beds.

Broad-based interest in a medical school continued for decades among citizens, politicians, and thought leaders in Austin. However, there was not a strong desire for a medical school from the leadership of UT Austin, who were concerned that a medical school would draw resources (including philanthropic support and state funds) away from the rest of campus. Within the UT System, many Regents, faculty, and staff worried that the establishment of an Austin medical school might also divert resources from existing UT medical schools. UTHSC–San Antonio supporters feared that resources could be reduced and the attention of patients, donors, and politicians diverted from San Antonio. In the case of UT Southwestern, these concerns existed, but an equally if not more important concern was that a medical school at UT Austin could eclipse UT Southwestern in reputation and research funding. UT Southwestern had distinguished itself as one of academic medicine's star campuses internationally, without the benefit of a research-intensive academic campus. A new research-intensive medical school, coupled with the substantial research capabilities of UT Austin, could potentially surpass what UT Southwestern had accomplished on its own. Yet there existed substantial resources and infrastructure to attract a medical school in Austin, including excellent hospitals, extensive residency training programs, good medical student clerkship experiences, and a long history of these significant resources in Central Texas. Let's examine some of these resources.

HISTORY OF BRACKENRIDGE HOSPITAL

Essential to the creation of a first-class medical school is an excellent teaching hospital: therefore, Brackenridge Hospital was pivotal to the creation of a medical school in Austin. As the oldest public hospital in Texas (Texas State Historical Association), it opened July 3, 1884, and was jointly owned by the City of Austin and Travis County until 1907, when the county withdrew its support. Initially, Brackenridge was called the City-County Hospital, but after Travis County withdrew, it became known as City Hospital. The hospital had cost $10,000 to build on a city block laid out in 1839, and it had a capacity of 40 patients. In 1915 a new, 45-bed hospital was built at the same site, and wings were added to reach an eventual bed capacity of 208.

In 1929, City Hospital was named after Robert J. Brackenridge, who led the campaign to finance the 1915 addition. During the 1970s, a 363-bed structure was built near the original building. The hospital was the site of Austin's first alternative birth center (1928), first intra-cranial surgery (1948), first intensive care unit (1960), first open-heart surgery (1961), and first cardiac care unit (1971). The Brackenridge emergency room became a level-one trauma center for the ten-county area. Brackenridge housed the area's first nursing school, established in 1915, and hosted the school until its transfer to the Austin Community College in 1984. The hospital became the principal home of medical residency training programs that developed in Austin. In 1995, the Seton Healthcare Family contracted to manage and operate Brackenridge Hospital.

SETON HEALTHCARE FAMILY

The mission of Seton is well demonstrated throughout its history. In 1897, a group of Austin women known as the St. Vincent's Aid Society became concerned that patients in the public hospital were not receiving appropriate religious and medical services. The Daughters of Charity of St. Vincent de Paul was established in the seventeenth century by

St. Vincent de Paul and St. Louise de Marillac in France. The group was dedicated to providing services to the sick and the poor. They are said to have been the first non-cloistered community of religious women to perform outreach in homes and on the streets as early as the 1630s.

In the United States, Elizabeth Ann Seton was a widow who established a religious community in Emmitsburg, Maryland, in 1809. The congregation was initially called the Sisters of Charity of St. Joseph's, and she became known as "Mother Seton." In 1810 the Sisters adopted the rules written by St. Vincent de Paul for the Daughters of Charity in France. St. Vincent's Aid Society asked this religious order to assist in developing a new hospital in Austin.

In 1898, the Daughters agreed to come to Austin if the Aid Society could provide a building and grounds suitable for a hospital. By 1900, the Aid Society raised the sum of $5,300. The money purchased Tobin Park, a five-acre tract on 26th Street between Nueces and Rio Grande in Austin. The State of Texas granted a charter to the Seton infirmary on April 4, 1900. The infirmary opened on May 29, 1902, and contained 17 private rooms, 11 wards, and facilities for the Sisters. Seton's first pamphlet said that the hospital "belongs to suffering humanity in general, irrespective of creed, color, nationality, financial standing, or any other limitation. All well-intentioned persons are cordially welcomed. True charity knows no bar to brotherhood."[11] The first Seton hospital in the region grew rapidly to 75 beds by 1914, and Seton now consists of over twenty hospitals and healthcare facilities across Central Texas. Among these was the Brackenridge Hospital, which Seton agreed to manage and operate for the City of Austin in 1995, pursuant to a thirty-year operating agreement. The management of the hospital was entirely consistent with the long-term mission of the Daughters of Charity, while simultaneously providing opportunities for medical education.

Engaging a Catholic organization (Seton) to run a public hospital presented complications in the provision of women's healthcare services, but the overall mission was well aligned with the goals of medical education. In 1997, the Vatican indicated that Seton must discontinue rendering healthcare services at Brackenridge Hospital that violated Catholic Ethical and Religious Directives. After considerable public concern in which a coalition of community groups opposed the elimination of women's health services at Brackenridge, Seton and the City of Austin reached an agreement in 2001. The City and, subsequently, the newly formed hospital district took back the fifth floor of Brackenridge Hospital and finished out its own women's hospital, described as a "hospital within a hospital." Within this twelve-bed acute care hospital, women could receive obstetrical, gynecological, and reproductive services regardless of their financial status, which was not under Seton's control or management. Shortly thereafter, in December 2003, the City and UT Medical Branch reached an agreement to operate the "hospital within a hospital" and to staff it with UT Medical Branch faculty, residents, and students. Amy Shaw Thomas, then the Vice Chancellor and Counsel for Health Affairs, was instrumental in addressing Regent Cyndi Taylor Krier's concerns that this arrangement might adversely affect UTHSC-San Antonio as a possible first step toward establishing a UTMB medical school regional campus in Austin. This arrangement continued until 2011, at which time the UT Medical Branch indicated it could not continue to operate the hospital within the limited budget provided by Central Health. As a consequence, the women's hospital was dissolved, and controversial reproductive services were no longer provided at Brackenridge Hospital but instead provided at St. David's Medical Center. Physicians and residents from UT Southwestern programs participated in care at St. David's for these purposes.

In April 2012, Seton reached an agreement with UT Austin and Central Health to build a new teaching hospital at UT Austin. Seton would construct, fund, own, and operate the new hospital. Central Health subsequently signed a sixty-year renewable lease with the UT System in October 2014 for use of the land upon which the hospital was built. Therefore, UT Austin leased the property to Central Health, and Central Health then subleased it to Seton so that the hospital district could ensure access to care for medically indigent Travis County residents. St. David's opposed the use of any public money for the new teaching hospital. No public money was used for this purpose.

On January 27, 2015, the Michael & Susan Dell Foundation (Dell Foundation) announced a gift of $25 million to name and partially fund the construction of the new teaching hospital on the UT Austin campus. The 211-bed Dell Seton Medical Center at the University of Texas became an integral part of the development of the new medical school at UT Austin and began accepting new patients in May 2017.

RESIDENCY TRAINING IN AUSTIN

Residency training is an essential part of a medical school. The first resident physicians appeared at Brackenridge Hospital in Austin in the 1930s. George Edmund Bennett, MD, was the first resident intern in 1931. The first resident in surgery was Claud Martin, MD, who started in 1932. Over the next decades, a significant number of interns and residents provided care to patients at Brackenridge. They were supervised by the hospital's general medical and specialty staff physicians. Brackenridge entered the national residency matching plan in July 1953. In this program, medical students listed their preferences for residency programs and were ranked by the programs to which they had applied. The students were then matched to the highest-ranked residency program that had accepted them. In 1955, the first of the current UT Austin residency programs was established in psychiatry.

In the 1960s, the Accreditation Counsel for Graduate Medical Education (ACGME) made the requirements for residency programs more stringent and required a full-time program director for each residency program. Medical specialty programs and freestanding internships without directors were phased out. Local physicians were concerned about the continuation of residency programs with the new requirements, as well as the availability of medical care for the indigent population.

In 1972, the Travis County Medical Society founded the Central Texas Medical Foundation (CTMF). The Foundation was organized with the following understanding:

- It would serve as a source of high-quality primary care physicians to serve the community both during and after physician training;

- Private physicians in the community would benefit from the presence of Graduate Medical Education (GME) and by their association with these teaching programs;
- Students would benefit from clinical training outside the university setting;
- The medical education program would assure the availability of high-quality primary care for the indigent population in Austin; and
- It would be the most effective interface for indigent care between its primary in-patient and out-patient care and access to specialty care.

Seton assumed the management and operations of Brackenridge Hospital on October 25, 1995, at which time the CTMF requested that Seton assume responsibility for the residency programs. Sponsorship for the not-for-profit CTMF was transferred from the Travis County Medical Society to Seton in 1996. Since that time, first UT Medical Branch, then UT Southwestern, and now Dell Medical School sponsored and developed residency programs in eighteen areas (appendix 1). During the consideration of the establishment of a medical school at UT Austin, UT had in excess of 200 residency positions in Austin, with a complement of faculty recruited to educate these residents.

Dr. James Lindsey is an alumnus of Harvard College and a graduate of the medical school at the University of St. Louis. He served as chief medical officer of the Seton Healthcare Family throughout the formative planning for the medical school. He was a clear leader in supporting residency and medical student education at Seton and, later, an important colleague with Sue Cox in creating successful programs there.

Initially, CTMF relationships were established with the UT Medical Branch and UTHSC-Houston. Rotating residencies were phased out in 1974; however, family medicine and transitional training programs were established in 1975. A freestanding program in general surgery was established as a three-year program until 1975, when it became a five-year program affiliated with St. Joseph's Hospital, in Houston. In 1980, these two programs became an integrated general surgery program. Obstetrics and gynecology also began in 1972 and was affiliated with the UT Medical Branch from 1972 until 1979 and affiliated with UTHSC-Houston from 1980 until 1990. In 1990 the CTMF obstetrics and gynecology training program was integrated with the program at St. Joseph's Hospital in Houston. The CTMF also had a pathology training program in the 1970s and early 1980s, when it was discontinued.

In 1996, all of the residency programs at Brackenridge became affiliated with the UT Medical Branch. On November 21, 2005, Seton and the UT Medical Branch reached a thirty-year agreement with a shared vision for the development of a UTMB Austin campus that supported the joint development of residency programs, undergraduate medical education, and biomedical research. Its goal was to double the number of medical residents over the next five years. In the fall of 2007, UTMB determined it would not develop a regional campus in Austin and would strategically refocus its attention on medical education programs in Galveston and the surrounding counties.

In October 2007, Executive Vice Chancellor Kenneth Shine and Vice Chancellor Amy Shaw Thomas discussed and evaluated which UT campus could most capably assume sponsorship of the UTMB medical education programs in Austin. Dr. Shine subsequently called UT Southwestern President Dr. Kern Wildenthal, who agreed that UT Southwestern would accept the transfer of the UT Medical Branch programs. At that time, both the UT System and the Austin community were seriously considering the possibility of a four-year medical school in Austin. Dr. Wildenthal, Dr. Shine, and Thomas studied the expansion and establishment of residency programs for up to 350 residents, along with the development of a small medical school. The study was premised on the understanding that neither legislative funding nor major financial commitments from UT Austin or UT Southwestern would be required. UT System leadership did consider making a significant capital investment in a new medical school in Austin during the spring of 2008. Community leaders also discussed and considered a substantial increase in the hospital district tax rate to support a new medical school in Austin.

Adverse economic conditions put the discussion of funding and planning a four-year medical school on hold in late 2008. However, UT Southwestern and Seton continued planning for the transfer and enhancement of the sponsorship of the existing UTMB residency programs in Austin to UT Southwestern, and the continuation of clinical rotations for third- and fourth-year UTMB medical students in Austin.

After more than a year of detailed, intensive negotiations, as described in detail below, UT Southwestern, the UT System, and Seton entered into an affiliation agreement outlining the expansion of residency programs in Austin, third- and fourth-year clerkships for UT Southwestern and UTMB medical students, and the development of a new Seton/UT Southwestern Center for Clinical Investigation. The affiliation agreement took effect in November 2009 and terminated in December 2014, due to the creation of the Dell Medical School.

UT SOUTHWESTERN RESIDENCY PROGRAMS

The negotiation of the affiliation agreement between Seton and UT Southwestern transferring UT Medical Branch medical education programs to UT Southwestern was a challenging one, yet it was particularly useful in preparing the groundwork for the eventual relationship between the new Dell Medical School and Seton. Key participants in these extensive negotiations were Dr. Kenneth Shine, Ms. Amy Shaw Thomas, and General Counsel Barry Burgdorf for the UT System; Charles Barnett and Greg Hartman for Seton; and President Daniel K. Podolsky and Dr. Sue Cox for UT Southwestern.

Kenneth I. Shine, MD, is a cardiologist and internist who served as Dean and Provost for the Health Sciences at the University of California, Los Angeles. He served two five-year terms as President of the Institute of Medicine of the National Academy of Sciences, now the National Academy of Medicine, in Washington, D.C., and was working in the aftermath of 9/11 at the Rand Corporation establishing the Center for Domestic and International Health Security. In the fall of 2003, a search committee chaired by Dr. Kern Wildenthal, the President of UT Southwestern, and consisting of the presidents of the other five health

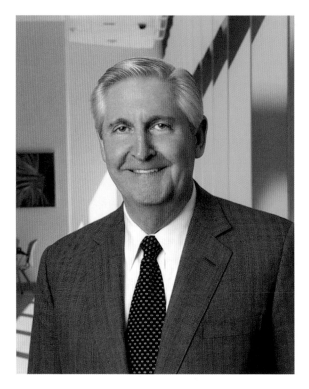

Kern Wildenthal

campuses, encouraged Shine to come to the UT System as the Executive Vice Chancellor for Health Affairs. Shine would be responsible for the six health institutions, including the four medical schools. During the interview process, Regent James Huffines asked Shine whether he would support the creation of a new medical school in Austin. Shine responded that he had no firm opinion on the subject, lacking detailed information about the needs and opportunities. Huffines then asked whether Shine had any objections to a medical school in Austin. Shine indicated that he had an open mind and harbored no such objections. The creation of two new medical schools, in Austin and South Texas, became a major focus of Shine's tenure as Executive Vice Chancellor.

Amy Shaw Thomas joined the UT System Office of Governmental Relations in January 1997 and the Office of Health Affairs at the UT System in September 2002. She later became Vice Chancellor for Academic and Health Affairs, Executive Vice Chancellor for Health Affairs, ad interim, and Senior Vice Chancellor for Health Affairs. Thomas previously worked as Legislative Counsel and Director of Debt Management and Public Policy for Senator Kay Bailey Hutchison when the latter was Texas State Treasurer. Thomas also served on the staff of a U.S. senator in Washington, D.C., and two members of the Texas Senate. She practiced public finance and general governmental law in the private sector. Thomas is a Phi Beta Kappa graduate of UT Austin with a BA with special honors in government and a Doctor of Jurisprudence from the University of Texas School of Law. She led negotiations and strategy on health initiatives, transactions, and affiliations on behalf of UT System institutions with their public and private partners. She played a continuing and substantial role in the planning, implementation, negotiations, and strategies related to the creation of the Dell Medical School and the UTRGV School of Medicine. As a longtime Austin resident, she had leadership roles on numerous prominent community boards and played a crucial role in addressing community interest in and support for a medical school in Austin. She was instrumental in the initiation of the community efforts led by Senator Kirk Watson.

A key leader in the overall efforts to obtain a medical school in Austin was Charles Barnett. Barnett was President and CEO of Seton. He started as an operating room technician in 1972, but as his career progressed, he became an executive in significant healthcare delivery organizations in Falls Church, Virginia, and Cincinnati, Ohio, prior to his arrival at Seton in Austin. With approximately thirty years of healthcare administration experience, Barnett joined Seton in 1993. He was a strong and persistent supporter of expanding medical education, particularly the growth of the graduate medical education programs with UT institutions, as previously described. Barnett strongly supported the development of undergraduate medical education and the concept of the medical school for Austin. He served as Chair of the Chamber of Commerce, the United Way for Greater Austin, and many other influential community organizations. He emphasized that the medical school would address the impending shortage of physicians in the region, pointing out the aging of the current physician population and the potential for many retirements. He also noted the ag-

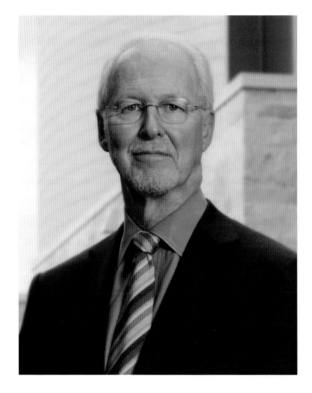

Charles Barnett

ing of the citizens in the region, overall growth of the population, and the opportunity to create a first-class medical school in collaboration with UT Austin. Barnett recognized the substantial economic advantages that a medical school would bring to Austin and Central Texas. During the final stages of efforts to obtain community support for the medical school in Austin, Barnett became the President of Healthcare Operations and the Chief Operating Officer of Ascension Health in St. Louis, the parent organization for Seton. He was particularly well positioned to advocate for the support of medical education in Austin and the construction of a new Seton-owned teaching hospital.

Greg W. Hartman had a number of positions in the Seton System during the 2003–2013 period in which the medical school developed. He was Senior Vice President for Marketing, Communications, and Planning, and Senior Vice President of Brackenridge Hospital, the critical teaching hospital for the UT medical education programs. During this interval, he also served as President and CEO of Seton Medical Center Austin. He was continuously involved in efforts to bring translational medical research and academic medicine to Central Texas, playing a key role in the negotiation of agreements to support GME programs between Seton and UT Southwestern, and subsequently between Seton, UT Austin, and the UT System to support both GME and undergraduate medical education programs. Hartman played a critical role in the impetus for Senator Watson's 10 Goals in 10 Years. Hartman's background as a strategic consultant for several political campaigns and his work with legislators in the Texas Senate and House, as well as with the former Texas State Comptroller John Sharp, prepared him well for these roles.

Hartman's role was a key one not only in inviting Senator Wat-

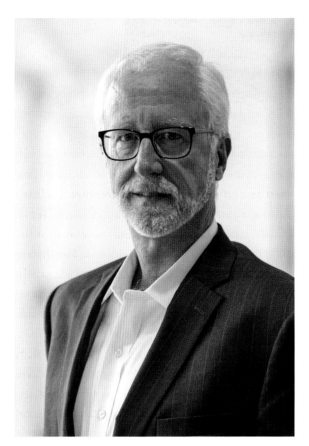

Greg Hartman

son to champion the creation of the medical school but also as a regular spokesperson for the benefits of a school and advocating for the passage of Central Health Proposition 1, which provided local property tax funding for the Dell Medical School.

Tim LaFrey played a key role in the Seton/UT System/UT Austin affiliation negotiations. LaFrey was an attorney and CPA who served in many leadership positions in charitable and professional organizations within Travis County and the state. He served as Executive Vice President for Common Strategy and Business Development for the Texas Ministry Market and oversaw hospital enterprise and insurance service divisions. He also served as Senior Vice President of Seton Ventures and Alliances for two years. LaFrey had served five years on the Seton Board of Trustees, chairing some of its key committees. His practical legal, business, and management expertise played a vital role in the successful negotiation and creation of partnerships and affiliations between Seton, the UT System, and UT Southwestern—and later Seton, UT Austin, and Central Health.

In addition to the support of the residents and the faculty to teach them, Seton also committed to the establishment of a clinical research institute with up to twenty faculty members. It committed to the recruitment of a director of the institute, which was accomplished the following year with the arrival of Dr. Steven Warach from the National Institutes of Health. Dr. Warach went on to develop important clinical programs in neurosciences and stroke.

A key element in contention during the negotiations was the desire of Seton to maintain complete control of all clinical and research programs in which UT Southwestern might become involved. The UT System was called upon to agree to these provisions as part of the negotiations. While provisions to give priority to Seton for certain clinical programs were approved, no control of research was approved.

SETON HEALTHCARE FAMILY LEADERSHIP

The leadership of Seton played a particularly important role in the establishment of the Dell Medical School at UT Austin and in mobilizing community support for the new school. Moreover, they firmly be-lieved that medical education was consistent with the mission of Seton. This particularly aligned with Seton's commitment to caring for medi-cally underserved individuals and populations. With the leadership of these and other administrators and the strong support of Seton's Board of Directors, substantial financial support was provided for medical residency programs and the clinical faculty to teach and supervise the residents. In addition, these clinical faculty, employed through a Seton nonprofit healthcare corporation, provided educational instruction to third- and fourth-year medical students. While the medical students were primarily from UT Medical Branch, there were also students from the Texas A&M College of Medicine and other institutions around the country who benefited from the clinical experiences provided by Seton and the clinical faculty.

When the opportunity arose in 2012 to obtain additional federal funding for care of the medically indigent, Seton worked closely with Central Health to create a mechanism that would allow both federal matching programs and their application to new services such as men-tal healthcare. That year, the Community Care Collaborative (CCC) was established as a public/private collaboration between Central Health and Seton for the provision of healthcare services to the uninsured and underinsured population of Travis County and to receive and distribute federal matching funds for Medicaid.

CHAPTER 3

CREATING THE IMPETUS

The Modern Era

Like the other University of Texas System medical schools, the creation of the school in Austin depended crucially on local support and action. Many individuals and organizations contributed to that effort. A brief description of some of these individuals and their contributions is described, most of whom will reappear as the story unfolds.

Frank Denius was a prominent attorney, philanthropist, and World War II military hero. He was also a distinguished alumnus of UT Austin. As early as the 1950s, Denius supported the development of a medical school at UT Austin. He believed that a world-class university required a world-class medical school. Creating a world-class university at his alma mater was his clear and deliberate goal. Denius lobbied many of his friends and colleagues to pursue this objective. In late 1957, the Mayor of Austin, Tom Miller, created a committee (of which Denius was a member) to bring a medical school to Austin. These citizens hoped to capitalize on the need for more physicians, and as resources became available in the aftermath of WWII, medical schools were being established across the country. Unfortunately for Austin, the citizens of San Antonio persevered in their cause to secure the next major medical school in the UT System. Denius continued his efforts over the next decades and paid particular attention to his relationship and interactions with James Huffines.

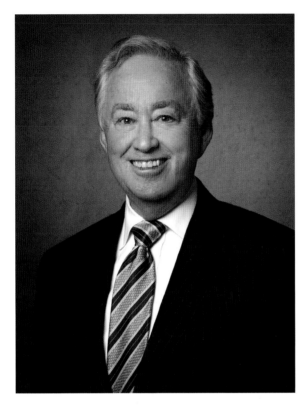

James Huffines

Huffines has had a distinguished career in business and banking, and played important roles in Texas politics. He served as the Appointments Secretary for Governor William P. Clements; served on a number of state, community, and business boards; and was a strong supporter and confidant of Governor Rick Perry. Perry appointed Huffines to the Board of Regents in February 2003 and reappointed him for a second consecutive term. He became Chair of the Board of Regents on June 2, 2004. Huffines was a leading citizen in Austin who was active in many community organizations and institutions. Not surprisingly, Denius regularly "whispered in his ear" about the possibility of a medical school at UT Austin.[1] Huffines earned a BA in finance from UT Austin in 1973 and understood and agreed with Denius's idea for a medical school in Austin. Huffines played a crucial role in the subsequent development of the medical school.

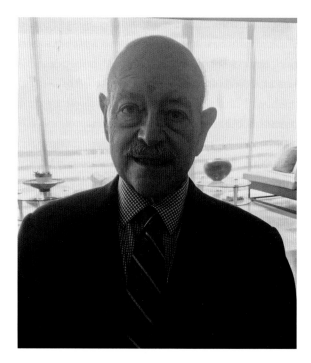

Mark Yudof

Mark G. Yudof was Chancellor of the UT System from August 1, 2002, to June 15, 2008. During this time, he played a significant role in the development of plans for the medical school in Austin. Yudof received his undergraduate degree at the University of Pennsylvania in 1965 and a law degree from the University of Pennsylvania School of Law in 1968. He joined the faculty at the University of Texas School of Law in 1971 and was Dean of the law school from 1984 to 1994. After three years as Executive Vice President and Provost at UT Austin, he served as President of the University of Minnesota from 1997 to 2002, when he returned to UT System as its Chancellor. He is a recognized expert in constitutional law, freedom of expression, and education law. As Chancellor, he quietly supported efforts to expand medical programs in Austin, including Shine's role as Executive Vice Chancellor.

Pete Winstead was the founding partner of Winstead PC. A distinguished attorney, he is a prominent community activist who has been repeatedly recognized by organizations in the city of Austin for his many meaningful contributions to the community. He was also counsel to the young entrepreneur Michael Dell, who was building a major computer technology company in Central Texas. Winstead worked on important projects for Dell, including taking Dell's company public. Winstead specifically recalls a United Way fundraising meeting in 2000 in which Dell asked him why Austin did not have a medical school. Dell's interest was driven by his growing company. He felt that an Austin medical school would significantly enhance his ability to recruit outstanding executives to his company. Dell was also increasingly interested in the health of children, stimulated by the commitment of his wife, Susan. Subsequently, Dell would provide philanthropic support for the Dell Children's Medical Center of Central Texas (Dell Chil-

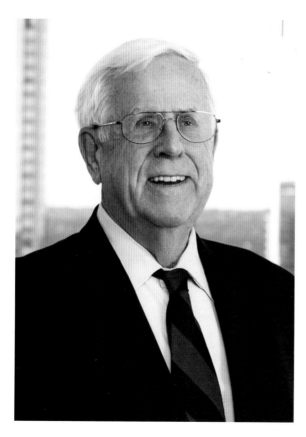

Pete Winstead

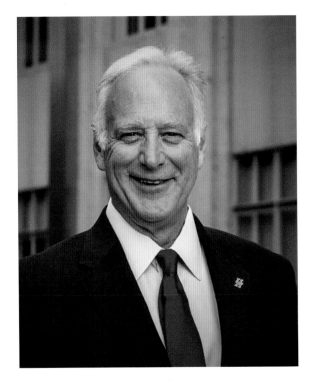

Kirk Watson

dren's Hospital) and eventually for the new medical school and teaching hospital, which would be named after him and his family.

State Senator Kirk Watson played a pivotal role in the creation of the Dell Medical School. Born in Oklahoma City, he grew up in Fort Worth, Texas, and received a bachelor's degree and JD from Baylor University in Waco. He served as Editor in Chief of the *Baylor Law Review* and graduated first in his law school class. After his clerkship with the United States Court of Appeals for the Fifth Circuit, he went into practice and eventually founded the Austin law firm of Watson Bishop London & Galow. He was President of the Texas Young Lawyers Association and was named the Outstanding Young Lawyer of Texas in 1994. Watson was elected Mayor of Austin in 1997 and was named the "best mayor in Texas for business" by *Texas Monthly Biz Magazine* in 1999. He was a popular mayor, reelected with 84 percent of the vote in 2000. Subsequently, he was elected to the Texas Senate in November 2006, with more than 80 percent of the vote. Watson was recognized by *Texas Monthly* as "Rookie of the Year" for the 2007 session, and in 2009 the magazine named him one of the state's ten best legislators. He received a number of awards and recognition for his leadership on a wide variety of issues, including the environment, business development, economic development, energy, and higher education. In 2009, he led the fight against a budget rider that would have effectively banned embryonic stem cell research at Texas universities. This strong background served the cause of the medical school extremely well, not only because of Senator Watson's outstanding reputation but also due to his political acumen, which would become crucial to the creation of the medical school. He publicly acknowledged that he was a cancer survivor. He was the author of the "10 Goals in 10 Years" proposal, which included starting a medical school at UT Austin. He was later President Pro Tempore of the Texas Senate.

Steve W. Leslie, PhD, played a central role in the development of the Dell Medical School, not only with the leadership of faculty on the UT Austin campus but also on the interface between the campus and the community. Leslie received undergraduate, master's, and doctoral degrees in pharmacology/toxicology from Purdue University. He joined the faculty of the College of Pharmacy at UT Austin in 1974. Leslie had a distinguished career as a research investigator, with approximately one hundred peer-reviewed scientific articles, and served as the program training director of an NIH training grant. He became Dean of the UT Austin College of Pharmacy in 1998. Leslie attributed his early interest in a medical school at UT Austin to the publication in November 1999 of the Institute of Medicine report *To Err Is Human: Building a Safer Health System*. Shine was President of the Institute of Medicine at the time and organized the effort to produce this report. Their mutual interests facilitated an easy and effective collaboration on the medical school project. In collaboration with colleagues, Leslie raised the funds to support a two-day symposium (November 29–30, 2000) entitled "Summit 2000: Better Medication Outcomes Through Healthcare Collaboration" (appendix 2). The summit brought together experts in the area of patient safety who highlighted the critical nature

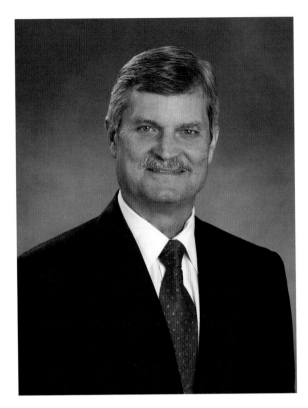

Steve Leslie

of interprofessional training and practice in controlling medical errors and increasing patient safety. Leslie became a major proponent of such interprofessional health education. He also became increasingly interested in the potential for commercialization of research products and the opportunity to enhance the commercial development of such products through incubators or other mechanisms in Central Texas.

Leslie became a member of the Board of the Central Texas Institute, which supported both of these initiatives. As a member of the Board, which is described in the next section, Leslie became acquainted with representatives of healthcare providers, hospitals, physicians, and others who shared his interests. This background served him well when he became Provost and Executive Vice President of UT Austin on January 15, 2007. His initial focus as Provost was on the importance of discovery, innovation, and its applications, as well as interprofessional education. Leslie repeatedly emphasized that a new medical school at UT Austin would require new funding, which he called "forever money"— that is, recurring funding so that the medical school's development would not impair the funding or development of the rest of UT Austin. He also supported opportunities for partnerships between UT Austin and the UT Health Science Center campuses, including UT Medical Branch and UT Southwestern. Subsequently, when an agreement was reached between UT Southwestern and Seton for the support of UT Southwestern residency programs in Austin at Seton facilities, Leslie regularly attended meetings of the Joint Conference Council (JCC) to oversee the affiliation between UT Southwestern and Seton.

Leslie was especially interested in the possibility of scientific collaborations between UT Austin and UT Southwestern. He saw the potential for the Dell Pediatric Research Institute (DPRI) and moved several research groups into that facility (to be discussed). His efforts in this regard were limited by the absence of any designated operating budget for the DPRI. During Leslie's tenure as Provost, Leslie and Shine convened a series of meetings to discuss in greater detail plans for a medical school with colleagues from UT Southwestern, including its President, Dr. Kern Wildenthal.

Leslie was determined to recruit an outstanding physician investigator to the UT Austin campus who might provide insight and leadership in the further development of education, research programs, and possibly a medical school. With the support of Science and Technology Acquisition and Retention (STARs) funding from the UT System's Office of Health Affairs and its Office of Academic Affairs, he recruited Dr. Robert O. Messing from the University of California, San Francisco. The STARs program provided UT PUF funding for construction, renovation, or equipment as part of campus recruitment packages for outstanding faculty. Leslie had previously been on a site visit of the Ernest Gallo Clinic and Research Center directed by Messing and had been impressed. It was Messing who later suggested to Leslie that Dr. S. Claiborne "Clay" Johnston, of the University of California, San Francisco faculty, would be an outstanding Founding Dean for a new medical school. Johnston would later become the Founding

Dean of the Dell Medical School. Messing provided important knowledge and insight into subsequent discussions about the medical school and worked very closely with Dr. Sue Cox in the initial establishment of the curriculum and facilities for the school.

Leslie's strong ties to the community were reflected in his 2011 appointment to the Chamber of Commerce Board of Directors. As Dean of the College of Pharmacy, Leslie encouraged the Chamber to think creatively about the potential for enhanced biotechnology companies in Austin, and he strongly supported the development of a research incubator and biotechnology incubator on the UT Austin campus. In January 2011, Leslie and Thomas made presentations to the Chamber of Commerce Board about the opportunities offered by the creation of a medical school in Austin. The presentations significantly increased the interest and enthusiasm of the Chamber of Commerce leadership in moving expeditiously to support the medical school. This level of enthusiasm of community groups led by the Chamber of Commerce stimulated Shine and Thomas to take action to build on this community interest. Leslie stepped down as Provost in October 2013 but continued to serve for another year as an adviser to the President of UT Austin on the development of the new medical school. Leslie was subsequently appointed Executive Vice Chancellor for Academic Affairs for the UT System in May 2015. He served in that role until October 2020.

Leslie was particularly effective when Central Health Proposition 1 was on the ballot in November 2012. Proposition 1 sought to increase the Central Health ad valorem tax rate of $0.05 per $100 valuation to improve healthcare in Travis County for a new medical school, consistent with the mission of Central Health. During the campaign for Proposition 1, Leslie, as well as Shine, Thomas, and Cox, regularly addressed community groups about the potential impact of a medical school on the campus, the community, and the nation. Thomas was a longtime member of the Downtown Austin Alliance (DAA) and the Austin Area Research Organization (AARO), and worked tirelessly to successfully garner support for a new medical school at UT Austin. UT leadership carefully avoided advocating in favor of Central Health Proposition 1 because political activities of this kind are forbidden for university employees. However, their educational discussions clearly helped those who wanted to understand the value of a new medical school in Austin and funding for the school through Central Health Proposition 1. In view of the historical reluctance of the President of UT Austin to support a medical school, Leslie's activities were particularly important.

CENTRAL TEXAS INSTITUTE

In late 2002, a group of educational institutions and health systems formed an association that was "committed to the advancement and application of healthcare education and biomedical research in Central Texas."[2] The members of the Central Texas Institute (CTI) included UT Austin, the UT Medical Branch, UTHSC-Houston School of Public Health, Seton, St. David's HealthCare Partnership, the Central Texas Veterans Health Care System, the Chamber of Commerce, and UTHSC–San Antonio. The CTI proposed an Austin academic health campus that would include programs such as (1) MD/PhD degrees, allied health sciences, nursing, and pharmacy education; (2) multi-institutional biomedical research; (3) education and research in public health and health policy; and (4) intellectual property for commercialization.

CTI's initial President was James C. Guckian, MD, the Executive Director of UT Medical Branch Austin Outreach, and previously Associate Vice Chancellor and interim Executive Vice Chancellor for Health Affairs at the UT System. Dr. Guckian made an important presentation to the Board of Regents on November 12, 2003, outlining the goals and objectives of the CTI (appendix 3).

Other officers included Dr. Thomas A. Blackwell, Associate Dean of Graduate Medical Education at UT Medical Branch (Vice President); Charles Barnett, President and CEO of Seton Healthcare Network (Treasurer); and Michael W. Rollins, President of the Greater Austin Chamber of Commerce (Secretary). Among the directors were Robert E. Askew Sr., MD, representing Austin physicians; Jon Foster, President and CEO of St. David's HealthCare Partnership; Anthony J. Infante, MD, PhD, Associate Dean for Research, School of Medicine,

UTHSC–San Antonio; Steve W. Leslie, PhD, Dean, UT Austin School of Pharmacy; Guy S. Parcell, PhD, Executive Dean, UTHSC-Houston School of Public Health; Robert W. Radlife, PhD, Acting Director, Central Texas Veterans Health Care System; Juan M. Sanchez, PhD, Vice President for Research, UT Austin Office of Research; Kenneth I. Shine, MD, Executive Vice Chancellor for Health Affairs, UT System administration; and Jerry S. Turner, JD, partner at Vinson & Elkins. Amy Shaw Thomas, JD, Vice Chancellor and Counsel for Health Affairs, was also an active participant in these meetings.

The officers and directors represented broad-based community interest in healthcare, research, and education in Austin, with representation from the two major hospital systems, UT Austin, the Chamber of Commerce, and other community leaders. A branch campus of the Houston School of Public Health was ultimately established at UT Austin consistent with the CTI goals. A joint MD/PhD program between UT Austin and the UT Medical Branch was also initiated. The CTI discussed and considered a variety of methods to support clinical trials and clinical investigations in Austin, though no systematic approach to these endeavors was established. Most members of CTI aspired to eventually have a medical school in Austin.

The CTI issued a public statement of its goals and objectives in September 2003 as interest in the medical school in Austin began to increase. The timing of this announcement was, in part, stimulated by Representatives Mike Krusee, R-Taylor, and Jack Stick, R-Austin, who proposed to secure funding for a biotechnology center with a medical school in Williamson County. This statement was one of numerous efforts intended to encourage the CTI and its members to create programs in Austin. The CTI continued to be a focus for conversation and ideas among the various parties interested in the continued development of medical education and research in Austin. Dr. Guckian facilitated a number of additional conversations between interested parties, including Pete Winstead, Gregory Weaver of Catellus Development Corporation (Catellus), the Department of Veterans Affairs (VA), and others.

Steve Leslie was Dean of the College of Pharmacy at UT Austin when the CTI was founded, and he became the Provost of UT Austin in 2007. His interactions with other members of the board of the CTI provided critically important background as efforts to create a medical school evolved over the subsequent decade. Leslie continued to work with a variety of organizations and leaders to facilitate medical education and research in Austin. He believed strongly in the mission of an academic health center but at first had to carefully navigate circumstances at UT Austin because the President and other key leaders did not initially support the creation of a medical school: they feared that it would draw key resources from other core campus functions.

The CTI's influence waned over the next several years as the UT System began to play a larger role in developing a medical school, but it provided an important forum for discussion between interested parties at a critical time.

UT AUSTIN PRESIDENT'S VIEWS

In April 2002, Larry Faulkner, the President of UT Austin, exchanged emails with James Guckian, who served as interim Executive Vice Chancellor for Health Affairs at the UT System. Faulkner articulated UT Austin's institutional goals as the following: "1) to increase the volume of health-related research in Austin in a way that will develop better opportunities for the faculty, 2) to create a better climate for stronger programs in nursing and pharmacy, 3) to develop a financial basis for special instrumentation that could strengthen Austin overall as a research center, 4) to create a basis for some strong MD/PhD programs, and 5) to possibly create opportunities for courses teaching the basic medical sciences so that we could support a large faculty in relevant areas."[3]

Faulkner examined four options to advance medical education and research in Austin. The first was to create a regional academic health center within UT Austin. "This model would be to create a structure like that found in many leading universities nationwide, such as UCLA, North Carolina, Michigan, and others."[4] He indicated a variant in which the UT Medical Branch became the partner responsible for medical education and clinical research, with possible appropriate partnerships with the VA and other hospitals. Although there were a number of positives with regard to this option, including UT's land, its national reputation, and units that might become part of a medical center such as nursing and pharmacy, there were also major negatives. Among these was that the "University of Texas at Austin has very little experience with the operation of medical programs."[5] Faulkner added, "This organizational scheme while common nationally, differs from that used by other medical centers in the UT System and even elsewhere in Texas."[6] There would be substantial statewide resistance to the expansion of UT Austin, particularly in general terms (the "Anyone but the Yankees" syndrome) and partly because the policy of the Board of Regents had been to build up other UT System institutions. There would be substantial resistance on campus to the dedication of resources in this direction, given the extensive discussions about the means of financing existing campus activities into the future.

Faulkner commented on a second option in which UT Medical Branch was the focus of leadership. There were many positives associated with this option, but he noted that negatives, political concerns in Austin, and internal resistance at the UT Medical Branch existed, based on a fear that resources from Galveston might be directed to Austin. A third possibility was to create a small, central organizational entity reporting to the Executive Vice Chancellor for Health Affairs at the UT System, who would be responsible for overseeing and coordinating a number of programs, including medical education and clinical research programs operated by the UT Medical Branch and research programs in the basic medical sciences conducted at UT Austin. Faulkner noted that it would be harder to get "coherent strategic development in this model and that UT System would incur some political exposure if and when it proposes a creation of a new health science component, even of this character."[7] In a fourth option, the Austin community could "create a non-profit central organizational entity reporting to its board and having essentially the same character of a cooperative academic health center."[8] Faulkner felt that creating this kind of new entity would also make it harder to get a coherent strategic direction and without the UT System, UT Medical Branch, or UT Austin directly in the name, it would be "harder to get the enterprise taken seriously in this state and nation."[9]

CONCEPT OF ACADEMIC HEALTH CENTER

On May 5, 2004, State Representative Jack Stick addressed the 500 attendees of the fourth-annual joint Real Estate Council of Austin luncheon. At that time, he provided a drawing of a medical school, pharmacy, nursing school, and medical office complex that could be built on the Robinson Ranch tract in Williamson County at an overall cost of $2 billion to $3 billion.

Stick's pronouncements stimulated Chancellor Yudof and Regent Huffines to request a statement from Shine about future developments in Austin. He prepared a white paper, entitled "Austin Academic Health Center Proposal" (appendix 4).

Shine shared the document with Charles Miller, Chair of the Board of Regents; Regent Rita Clements, who chaired the Health Affairs Committee of the Board of Regents; and Regent Cyndi Taylor Krier, who had a particular interest in medical school developments in Austin that might affect the UT medical school in San Antonio. The white paper was approved by Chancellor Yudof and was "acceptable" to Jack Stobo, then President of the UT Medical Branch, and Larry Faulkner, then President of UT Austin. Regent Huffines expressed great interest in the plan and was supportive of the draft. The white paper recapitulated many elements of the Executive Vice Chancellor's presentation to the Board of Regents, at the August 2004 board meeting (appendix 5).

The Shine white paper described the status of health education, research, and patient care in the Austin area. It outlined a set of principles around which an academic health center might be developed. These included an enterprise of the "highest quality so as to recruit a world-class faculty and develop outstanding educational and clinical programs that are nationally recognized." The academic health center should be physically proximate to the UT Austin campus, with the former Mueller airport site being one such location. Shine recommended an incremental approach that would include the creation and staffing of two or more research institutes, as well as the gradual expansion of educational programs for undergraduate students seeking an MD or MD/PhD program, and the addition of postgraduate training programs in various medical specialties. The white paper proposed the establishment of a medical research institute headed by a director who reported to the President of the UT Medical Branch for operations, and the presidents of the UT Medical Branch and UT Austin with regard to program development. Faculty could have joint appointments at UT Medical Branch and UT Austin. It was noted that Seton was about to build and open a children's hospital and related medical office building at the former Mueller airport site, with a goal of completion in 2007, which was met. The Central Texas Veterans Health Care System also expressed interest in building an inpatient/ambulatory facility on the site (which did not occur).

The white paper suggested that the first two years of medical school might be provided to a group of UTMB students educated at UT Austin by "a combination of teachers in the research institute, scientists at UT Austin, and well-trained physician teachers from the various affiliated teaching hospitals." Fifty to sixty UTMB students were already being educated in Austin during their third and fourth years of medical school. There was a discussion of current and future residency programs, the establishment of a regional campus of the UTHSC-Houston School of Public Health, and expanded programs to provide care to indigent patients. It was suggested that "over the course of 10 to 12 years, development of a critical mass of resources might allow the establishment of a new medical school. Accreditation for such a unit could be as part of UT Medical Branch. In this organizational structure the dean of the medical school would report to the president of UT Medical Branch and have a programmatic relationship to the president of UT Austin."

Dr. Shine proposed a hypothetical work plan that included the development of an academic health center site—for example, the former Mueller airport in the period from 2004–2006. During this time, additional residency programs would be developed, the number of medical students participating in clerkships in Austin hospitals during their third and fourth years at UTMB would increase, and funding would be sought for a research institute with major contributions from private sources. The overall work plan suggested that the period from 2006–2009 would include the development of the MD/PhD program, expanded VA activities, and further recruitment of faculty. In the period 2007–2008, a second research institute would be started, funded primarily from private sources, and followed by the recruitment of a director and faculty for the second institute. From 2010–2012, the number of medical students would continue to expand, and basic science courses for medical students in their first two years would be conducted in Austin. "Additional funding would be obtained for expanded instruction including classrooms of smaller group instruction, auditoria, and learning labs." In 2014, the first class would be admitted to an Austin medical school, which would continue as part of UT Medical Branch, but with a programmatic relationship in reporting to the President of UT Austin. No formal written responses to the white paper were made by the Board of Regents; however, the correspondence led to a formal presentation to the Board in August 2004. That presentation was quietly well received by the Regents.

ECONOMIC IMPACTS
THE GREATER AUSTIN CHAMBER OF COMMERCE

For decades Austin had been best known for UT Austin, whose student body eventually exceeded 50,000, as well as the Texas state government, Bergstrom Air Force Base, and its banks. In the 1970s, a number of high-tech corporations, including IBM, Texas Instruments, and Tracor, began to relocate to or expand in Austin. In 1987, the Sematech Consortium, which was intended to advance the U.S. chipmaking industry, and Michael Dell's computer company began to grow and anchor the Central Texas economy. Shortly after Dell's conversation with Winstead about the need for a medical school in Austin, the Chamber of Commerce undertook a more vigorous effort to attract new companies, led by businessmen including Gary Farmer, owner of Heritage Title Company; Joe Holt, a banking executive; Michael W. Rollins, President of the Chamber; Senator Watson; Charles Barnett; Winstead; and a number of other community leaders. Chamber leaders designed a corporate recruitment and economic development strategy that became known as "Opportunity Austin." In its original publication in 2003, an emphasis was placed on "medical products."[10] The initiative was designed to focus on "stages" of the bioscience development process as local economic niches. However, the report recognized that "because Austin is at a disadvantage compared to many other major metros due to lack of a medical school and only one local teaching hospital, it is unlikely that the region will be able to develop an exhaustive infrastructure for medical R&D and testing."[11] This economic development effort increased the interest in the business community in establishing a medical school in Austin. Subsequently, the Chamber of Commerce became increasingly active in its support of a medical school. It later commissioned an economic analysis of the impact of a medical school on the region.

TEXAS PERSPECTIVES, INC. (TXP) REPORT: OPPORTUNITY AUSTIN

Opportunity Austin, the activity of the Chamber of Commerce designed to stimulate the recruitment and expansion of businesses across the region, commissioned a study by TXP (President Jon Hockenyos) in early 2006 "in evaluating the current and potential economic impact of Austin's primary medical sector."[12] The report, which was released in August 2006, concluded that hospitals and ambulatory medical services during 2005 accounted for "$8.9 billion in total regional output, $3 billion in earnings, and supported 85,466 jobs in the Austin metro area."[13] The report went on to conclude that "if Austin would have matched the national average (7.1% of the area employment base, compared to 5.7% in Austin last year) then the total impact would be significantly larger, creating an additional $2.3 billion in output, $820.1 million in earnings, and 22,175 more jobs."[14] The report went on to state, "Close proximity to high-quality medical service, especially a hospital, is consistently cited as a top site selection factor for expanding and relocating businesses. At the same time quality of life is assuming an increasing role in attracting both business and residents, with healthcare at full capacity (both in terms of access and quality) obviously an important consideration."[15] In the report, TXP reviewed current ambulatory hospital activities in the greater Austin area. This included both direct activity and "indirect effects" produced by the healthcare industry in the community. It reviewed both current activities and plans by major healthcare providers for expansions and new facilities.

STICK/KRUSEE PROPOSAL

As previously noted, in the fall of 2003, actions by two Central Texas legislators stimulated serious interest in a medical school for Central Texas. State Representatives Mike Krusee, R-Taylor, and Jack Stick, R-Austin, indicated that they would attempt to obtain legislative support during the 2005 session to secure funding for a biotechnology center with "a medical school at its foundation."[16] It was estimated that they would seek $100 million to $200 million in initial funding and proposed that the Robinson Ranch tract in northern Travis County and southern Williamson County would be an ideal location for the biotech center. Shortly thereafter, Stick provided an artist's diagram of what a biotechnology center might look like, including the medical school. Charles Barnett, then Chair of the Chamber of Commerce, indicated that it might be too early to conclude that the area needed a medical school. Early in 2004, the newly appointed Executive Vice Chancellor Shine indicated to Krusee that locating a medical school so far from the main Austin campus would be problematic. Krusee and Stick continued to advocate for this development, but no significant funding was obtained during the 2005 session.

THE PERRYMAN REPORT

In 2007, the Chamber of Commerce commissioned a report on the potential for a major medical school in Austin from the Perryman Group. Ray Perryman is a well-known economist in Texas who produced a report in April 2007 entitled *The Impact of Developing a Major Medical School at the University of Texas at Austin on Regional and State Business Activity*. Perryman indicated that "in addition to the potential in advancement in human health and well-being, the presence of a major medical school offers tremendous economic benefits for the area where it is located. It can bring substantial gains and business activities through its operations, student spending, and other activities; foster research in a broad area of sciences associated with healthcare; and contribute to the development of areas such as the life sciences."[17] Perryman pointed out that "the greatest gains tend to occur in locations which combine a major research university with a large medical school."[18]

Among the major findings of the report were the following: "The joint presence of the excellent scientific research programs at the University of Texas at Austin with a major medical school would greatly expand competitiveness in this area. The Perryman Group estimates that ongoing operations of a major medical school in Austin would generate some $2.381 billion in yearly spending in the regional economy ($2.917 billion in the state) and (19,307 jobs, 21,484 in the state)."[19] The report went on to state that "the enhanced healthcare outcomes which may reasonably be expected may also likely generate more than $11 billion annually in net social benefits."[20] The highlights concluded, "The University of Texas medical school in Austin could be the central factor in positioning Texas more prominently as a competitor for biosciences cluster in improving the health and well-being of all the state's citizens."[21] The report provided information about the impact of research-intensive medical schools across the United States. It outlined the advantages of an Austin-area location for a medical school, including "the wealth of knowledge and research capacity already in place at the University of Texas at Austin and the presence of outstanding local hospitals, such as Seton and St. David's."[22] Perryman noted, "Austin is also a significant center for electronics, software, and several other technology sectors as well as notable private research entities. Many local firms and other enterprises are engaged in activities which have enormous potential for commercialization in conjunction with future health-related advances and applications."[23] Perryman detailed many specific advantages of a relationship with UT Austin, with its very comprehensive science, engineering, and technology programs, and provided detailed descriptions of the medical facilities in the community.

The Perryman report asserted the important economic impact of a medical school, including jobs and financial benefits that would be synergistic with efforts to improve health and well-being. All of this was consistent with the interest of the Chamber of Commerce in supporting a medical school in the city and provided important justification for its continued efforts in this regard.

TRAVIS COUNTY HEALTHCARE DISTRICT (CENTRAL HEALTH) STRATEGIC PLAN

On January 5, 2007, Central Health published a strategic plan with a vision for "Central Texas as a model healthy community." It emphasized enhancing the health of residents, promoting an integrated healthcare system that was transparent to consumers, and providing improvements in access to quality healthcare and improvements that tied payments for healthcare services to measurable performance. A major goal was the integration and improvement of Travis County's indigent care system. The plan identified the need for specialty services for medically indigent patients, including a specific goal to "implement a community-wide effort including private physicians, hospitals, and University of Texas Medical Branch at Galveston to agree on an approach to address the lack of system capacity for care."[24]

AUSTIN AREA RESEARCH ORGANIZATION (AARO) ECONOMIC ASSESSMENT

AARO describes itself as a "non-partisan, non-profit organization that builds on the savvy and brain power of 110 leaders from the Central Texas region." Its stated mission is "AARO engages regional leaders in data-driven deliberative action to enhance the long-term economic and social well-being of Central Texas." AARO had a long-standing interest in medical education in Texas and the development of a medical school in particular. It served as an important platform for exchanging ideas in these areas. In 2008–2010, AARO expressed increased interest and enthusiasm for an Austin medical school, which encouraged community discussions about such a project. Amy Shaw Thomas was an active AARO member who served as the primary advocate with AARO in the discussions about a medical school.

After the profound economic downturn of the U.S. and Texas economies in 2008, AARO commissioned another study in 2011 by TXP on life sciences in the region and their future potential, titled *Academic Medicine in Austin: Economic Implications.* The report identified Austin as "emerging as a best-in-class sciences community with over 7,000 employed in the industry. There are over 57,000 working in the healthcare industry."[25] The report went on to state that "the convergence of biology and technology allows Austin to capitalize on its global reputation as a technology hub."[26] TXP described past, present, and future opportunities in the life sciences area. It reviewed successful science parks across the country and listed the attributes of these activities.

In a section of the report entitled "Academic Medicine in Austin" and subtitled "Economic Impact," TXP stated, "Austin based efforts ultimately could have close to 5,000 physicians, faculty, and associate staff."[27] TXP estimated that this would generate about $600 million in direct annual economic activity. The report continued: "Academic medicine should also stimulate further activity in the local life sciences cluster. Research by the Milburn Institute suggested that an additional 2,100 jobs and $340 million in direct annual activity could be attributed to the full implementation of academic medicine."[28] The TXP report concluded that the combination of efforts in health and academic medicine could produce over $1 billion to $2 billion in additional earnings and around 7,000 permanent jobs. "When the ripple effects are considered, the impact doubles. $2 billion in activity and approximately 15,400 permanent jobs."[29] This report produced somewhat different numbers than previous studies but again emphasized the profound potential opportunities and impact that expanded academic medical programs would have on the community. It provided important background information that supported later efforts to raise taxes to fund a medical school in Austin.

THE HOCKENYOS REPORT

A later economic study was done in August 2012 by TXP, whose principal was Jon Hockenyos. This report was prepared as part of the campaign and support for Central Health Proposition 1. Hockenyos estimated that "the impact of the combination of the medical complex and economic development in the life sciences translates into a total of almost $1 billion (in 2012 dollars) in direct annual spending and about 6,900 direct jobs. When the ripple effects are factored in, the impact rises to a total annual economic impact of about $2 billion in economic activity, almost $905 million in earnings, and 15,400 jobs in the Austin area."

COMPETING PROJECTS

Round Rock, Texas, became a focus for expanding medical education programs during the first decade of the twenty-first century. St. David's Round Rock Medical Center completed an expansion in 2006. Scott & White Healthcare opened a hospital in Round Rock in 2007, and Seton Medical Center Williamson also opened in Round Rock in 2008. Also in 2008, Texas A&M opened a building there that housed certain of its health science center functions and provided rotations for approximately 50 third- and fourth-year medical students.

Both St. David's School of Nursing at Texas State University and Austin Community College offered health science programs at Round Rock campuses. It was clear that Texas A&M hoped to develop a medical school in Central Texas through its Round Rock campus. Although the Texas Legislature appropriated funds to Texas A&M for an academic building in Round Rock, the resources available to the campus were very limited. Moreover, hospitals in the region did not support Texas A&M residency programs, primarily because Texas A&M favored primary care residency programs, and the hospitals preferred and needed specialty training. Although there was considerable public discussion and publicity about a potential medical school at Round Rock, it was clearly a limited expansion of the existing Texas A&M College of Medicine, whose primary campus was in Temple, in conjunction with Scott & White Hospital. The establishment of the Texas A&M Health Science Center in Round Rock had little to no effect on plans to create a medical school in Austin.

CHAPTER 4

AUSTIN'S NEXT STEPS

Some Key Players

While support for the medical school in Austin was growing, a key component of its actual development was the involvement of the UT Medical Branch in Austin. Many of the physicians in Austin and Central Texas had been educated at the UT Medical Branch and were supportive of the efforts of their alma mater. The clinical and educational activities and programs of the UT Medical Branch were largely conducted on Galveston Island and the areas immediately contiguous to it. The population on Galveston Island was fairly limited for a medical school, but the John Sealy Hospital had done well throughout the years because medically indigent patients from all over the state were routinely sent there. As a result of the growth of public hospitals in other parts of the state and the presence of medical schools in most of the metropolitan areas, referrals to the hospital diminished significantly in the 1980s and 1990s. The Texas Legislature was increasingly reluctant to provide substantial appropriations to UT Medical Branch to fulfill its indigent care mission. The leadership of the UT Medical Branch looked to Austin to expand its educational and clinical programs, and to seek research opportunities. UT Medical Branch President Jack Stobo initially led these efforts.

John D. "Jack" Stobo, MD, is a nationally recognized rheumatologist who served as President of the UT Medical Branch from 1997

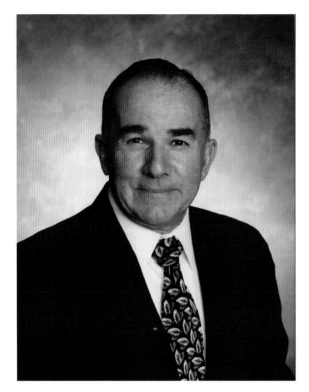

John D. "Jack" Stobo

to 2007. He previously had a distinguished career as the William Os-
ler Professor of Medicine and Physician-in-Chief of the Johns Hopkins Hospital. From 1976 to 1985, Stobo served as head of the Section
of Rheumatology and Clinical Immunology at the University of California, San Francisco, where he was also an investigator at the Howard
Hughes Medical Institute. As President of the UT Medical Branch, he
recognized that the institution could not reach its full potential if it was
limited principally to Galveston Island.

The patient population was not adequate for the diversity of resources required to support the most outstanding clinical programs on
Galveston Island. The financial foundation for the medical school in
Galveston could not rely on the population of the Island, which num-
bered approximately 65,000 at that time. In addition to exploring options for the medical school to expand north toward Houston, Stobo

recognized that opportunities in Austin were attractive. He supported the development of MD/PhD programs involving UT Medical Branch and UT Austin to advance educational and research opportunities. For clinical programs, Stobo envisioned the possibility of Austin becoming a regional campus of the UT Medical Branch. Residency programs between Seton and the UT Medical Branch were developing satisfactorily. Seton was also investing in its pediatric programs and had plans to build a freestanding pediatric hospital. Pediatrics was one of the areas with a very limited patient population on Galveston Island, and the UT Medical Branch had specific expertise in the area. UTHSC–San Antonio had set a precedent for the development of a regional academic health center in the Lower Rio Grande Valley with facilities and programs in those communities. Austin might provide an opportunity for such a regional academic health center (appendix 6).

The commitment of the UT Medical Branch to the expansion of programs in Austin was reflected in the appointment of Dr. T. Samuel Shoemaker, Dean of UT Medical Branch Regional Programs in Austin, on July 14, 2006. Shoemaker completed an internship in surgery and residency in anesthesiology before joining the faculty at the University of Utah, where he was a Professor in the Department of Anesthesiology and Associate Dean for Curriculum and Minority Affairs. Subsequently, he moved to the University of Hawaii, where he served as the Dean of the John A. Burns School of Medicine. In the announcement of his appointment, UT Medical Branch medical school Dean Valerie M. Parisi indicated that "we have been developing a network of collaborations in Austin since the 1950s, when UT Medical Branch medical students first began doing rotations in this state's capital city. Today there are vigorous partnerships in Austin, the Seton Healthcare Family and Central Texas Veterans Administration (to name just a few) that form the foundation for our future activities in the region."[1] She went on to say that Shoemaker "will be an innovative leader who will share the vitality and growth of the Austin programs and forge even stronger alliances among the Seton Healthcare Family, UT Austin, UT Medical Branch, and the greater Austin community."[2] Shoemaker became active in recruiting additional faculty to UT Medical Branch programs in Austin. He was an articulate spokesperson for expanding educational and research programs in the area. On a number of occasions, he made reference to the potential for a regional campus of the UT Medical Branch that might expand into a full-fledged medical school in Austin. At times, his public statements caused concern with the leadership of the UT System because they went beyond the commitments of the Board of Regents. However, he did forge important partnerships with community organizations in support of education and academic medicine in the region. Shoemaker's role changed substantially when the residency programs were transferred to UT Southwestern in 2009 (to be described in greater detail), and he then became a Chancellor's Health Fellow at the UT System's Office of Health Affairs. During his tenure in Austin, he also served as President of the CTI, which was previously described. On July 23, 2010, Shoemaker was named Dean of the medical college at Texas A&M.

Key senior members of the UT System staff supported President Stobo's expansion efforts in Austin. Programmatic development was supported especially by Kenneth I. Shine, MD, who had recently been recruited to the UT System, and by Amy Shaw Thomas, who served in many leadership roles at the UT System. Shine and Thomas worked very closely together to support and advance the expansion of medical education activities of UTMB and UT Southwestern, as well as, eventually, the development and creation of the new medical school, including the negotiations of key partner and funding agreements.

Vice Chancellor Randa Safady also played a crucial role at several steps in the process, especially in philanthropic developments. Safady was the UT System Vice Chancellor for External Relations during the development of the Dell Medical School. A graduate of Texas State University (formerly Southwest Texas State University), she earned a PhD in higher education administration from UT Austin. After holding several positions at St. Edward's University, she led a major philanthropic enterprise for UT Austin until she was appointed Vice Chancellor for External Relations for the UT System in 2003. She was responsible for many innovations, including a PBS series, *State of Tomorrow*, and played a key

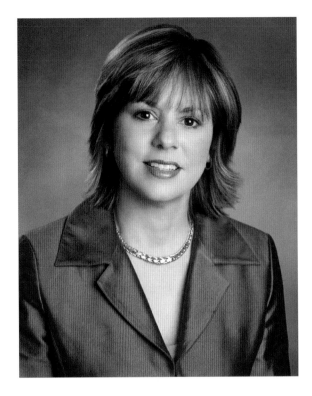

Randa Safady

role in achieving the funding for the DPRI as a first step toward the Dell
Medical School. She also consulted with other institutions, including
Seton, in coordinating efforts for philanthropic support after the successful vote to enable Central Health to provide financial support for
the medical school.

DELL PEDIATRIC RESEARCH INSTITUTE (DPRI)

Shine arrived as Executive Vice Chancellor in November 2003. On
March 15, 2004, Pete Winstead met with Shine at the Headliners Club
in downtown Austin, and Winstead told Shine of his relationship with
Michael Dell and outlined Dell's interest in a medical school in the city.
Winstead also indicated that he would be pleased to introduce Shine

to the Executive Director of the Dell Foundation, Janet Mountain, so that they could discuss ways to move toward the creation of a medical school in Austin. Shine suggested a strategy to start slowly and incrementally with a series of research initiatives. Seton was building a pediatric hospital at the former Mueller airport site, where land might be available to build a facility dedicated to pediatric research. Shine suggested that the Board of Regents might become more comfortable with the creation of a medical school in Austin if the initial focus was on the development of the pediatric research institute. Winstead encouraged Shine to pursue this approach.

As previously observed in the communications between President Larry Faulkner of UT Austin and Dr. James Guckian at CTI, there was reluctance on the UT Austin campus to vigorously pursue the creation of a medical school, which might divert important resources, including philanthropy, away from general campus needs. At the same time, there were serious reservations among the Board of Regents, particularly those from cities with existing UT health campuses.

In a November 2003 article published in the *Austin American-Statesman*, Rita Clements, a Dallas Regent and Chair of the Health Affairs Committee of the Board of Regents, and Cyndi Taylor Krier, a former State Senator who was a UT System Regent from San Antonio, said, "They want to be sure existing schools are adequately funded and collaborating as much as possible. I don't think it's good for Austin, I don't think it's good for South Texas, and I don't think it's good for El Paso, for this to become a tug of war," Krier said.[3] Clements said: "In light of state budget cuts, the future school for Austin is way down the line."[4]

After the Shine conversation with Pete Winstead, further discussions with President Jack Stobo of UT Medical Branch, and a very preliminary outreach to the Dell Foundation, Regent Huffines and Shine thought it was appropriate to make a presentation to the Board of Regents. To this point, several Regents had been very reluctant to see UT System discussions of an Austin medical school. Shine and Chancellor Yudof met with Rich Oppel, the Editor of the *Statesman*, in a briefing on education in Austin. This was reflected in a commentary in the *States-*

man (June 20, 2004) describing Shine's vision for a medical school. This resulted in an immediate statement of concern by Krier, the Regent from San Antonio. Yudof promptly assured Krier that Shine had communicated no such vision, which was the case. Shine did make a presentation on August 11, 2004, and did not explicitly discuss the establishment of a medical school in Austin, instead focusing on the concept of an Austin academic health center built substantially on UT Medical Branch activities. He described opportunities for substantially expanding health science research, education, and patient care in Austin. Shine reviewed the long-standing and substantial commitment of the UT Medical Branch in Austin (appendix 5). This included the education and rotation of as many as one hundred UT Medical Branch medical students through Austin hospitals and clinics. The prominent nature of existing residency programs, the new women's hospital at Brackenridge operated by the UT Medical Branch, the joint MD/PhD program between the UT Medical Branch and UT Austin, and the development of a state-of-the-art imaging program between the Central Texas Veterans Administration, the UT Medical Branch, and UT Austin were all examples of successful foundational activities of the UT Medical Branch in Austin.

Shine emphasized that many other opportunities existed and proposed that an academic health center be developed "in accordance with the following principles."[5] These principles included a commitment to the highest-quality health enterprise, which would proceed in a stepwise fashion and only with adequate funding. This included an incremental approach to increase programs for undergraduate students seeking MD or MD/PhD degrees and the addition of new residency training programs. Among the principles was the potential establishment of one or more medical research institutes that would capitalize on synergies between UT Austin and the UT Medical Branch. The UT Medical Branch would continue to expand its collaborative programs with institutions in Austin as part of specific institutes. Other schools, including UTHSC–San Antonio and Texas A&M, would be encouraged to enter into collaborations in medicine, nursing, pharmacy, allied health, and other areas of these institutes. UTHSC-Houston would continue to develop collaborations with UT Austin in research and education (ultimately resulting in a School of Public Health regional campus at UT Austin).

Shine's presentation indicated the contributions these programs would make for the care of the medically indigent and the significant potential for economic development in the region. It was noted that the City of Austin was prepared to set aside fifteen acres of the former Mueller airport site to UT for research and educational purposes proximate to the new Dell Children's Hospital. Shine suggested that this property might "form the initial location of the educational, research, or clinical facilities central to developing an academic health center."[6] He further identified the importance of local community support, including philanthropy, and reiterated the need for private support for expanding the academic health center. Shine concluded that the expansion of medical education in Austin would require effective public-private synergies and support from the local community. He indicated that there seemed to be a convergence of interest and opportunity to build on.

The Board of Regents took no immediate or specific action from Shine's presentation; however, several Regents, including those from cities with established health science center campuses, indicated that the approach was appropriate and that they were supportive of these efforts. Chair Huffines, Chancellor Yudof, and Shine concluded that proceeding in these directions was sensible.

THE FORMER MUELLER AIRPORT SITE: THE CITY OF AUSTIN

The Robert Mueller Municipal Airport operated from 1930 to 1999 as the principal airport in Austin. Located a few miles northeast of downtown Austin, it was named for Robert Mueller, a member of the city council who died while in office in January 1927. There were numerous discussions in Austin about relocating the Mueller airport as airline traffic increased. After the Bergstrom Air Force Base, located southeast of downtown Austin, closed as an active military base in 1993 and was decommissioned as a reserve base in 1996, the City of Austin moved the Mueller airport to the former base in 1999.

The 711 acres of the former Robert Mueller Municipal Airport stood unused for over half a decade before the City of Austin approved a development plan for its use. After prolonged community and political discussions, with substantial input from neighborhood groups, the Mueller Community was developed by Catellus (whose parent company was ProLogis). The project is a mix of residential, commercial, and retail developments with designated parks and green space. There is a large commercial center bordering Interstate 35. One of the earliest occupants of the Mueller community was Dell Children's Hospital, a thirty-two-acre campus with 170 patient beds and a total of 1,400 employees. It was the first acute-care facility in the world to achieve LEED Platinum certification, a designation that was also sought for UT Austin buildings on the development. Dell Children's Hospital has undergone significant expansion, and a thirty-bed Ronald McDonald House was built near the hospital.

In 2004, as discussions continued about the development of a medical school in Austin, the City of Austin offered a fifteen-acre site of the Mueller Development to UT for a new medical school. These rumors stimulated an initial meeting between the Mueller Neighborhoods Coalition (Coalition) and the leadership of the CTI, which was advocating for a Central Austin location for a medical facility. Shortly thereafter, a series of meetings occurred between the Coalition and the leadership of the UT System and UT Medical Branch. These included meetings during February, April, May, June, and August of 2005. As the conversations developed, there was increasing support among the Coalition for the use of the fifteen-acre site for the development of medical facilities. Subsequent discussions suggested that UT Austin may need increased acreage, and the university explored the purchase of an additional ten acres, bringing the total to nearly twenty-seven acres. The Coalition, under community activist Jim Walker's leadership, identified a series of concerns. In priority order, these included:

1. That the UT presence at Mueller regardless of use shall never exceed the twenty-five-acre total in the proposal under consideration. The Coalition also stated that they believed that land acquisition by UT adjacent to or near Mueller must comply with the relevant neighborhood plan adopted by the City of Austin, and that compliance was to be based on UT's good-faith efforts working with the relevant neighborhoods.

2. That the Capital Area Health Education Center would expand its operations and its working relationship with community leaders in East Austin. This included an expansion of UT-supported health services in the region, which would particularly benefit lower-income residents and their health needs.

3. That UT would seek opportunities to support the availability of affordable housing at Mueller, as it would possibly benefit UT faculty, employees, and students at various income levels involved with the proposed facility.

4. That UT would work in good faith with all relevant City of Austin neighborhood teams related to private businesses desiring to locate near the facilities.

It was emphasized that all buildings on the site would have to meet the Mueller Development design guidelines and be consistent with the surrounding Mueller redevelopment. The Coalition indicated that it understood that UT facilities would consist of academic and medical research uses, including outpatient clinics, i.e., a possible VA clinic, and that UT would not build a new hospital.

The Coalition went on to identify that "a UT presence at Mueller would be the core location of a network of health-related facilities, for example, an academic imaging center at one of the downtown hospitals. Therefore, we believe that UT would significantly benefit from the expansion of the Capital Metro Transit System, specifically commuter rail or other modes of fixed guideway transit. As a reminder, the Mueller Master Plan is a transit-oriented development to potentially maximize the provision of real or alternative shared lanes modes of travel. Meaning we need rail extensions to Mueller as soon as possible."[7]

NEIGHBORHOOD INTERACTIONS

In December 2004, word began to spread that the UT System and UT Medical Branch would be interested in locating the beginnings of an academic health center on the Mueller site. Shine had a series of meetings with representatives of local community groups regarding these developments. A major player in the relationship with neighborhood groups regarding the background and approval of the DPRI was Jim Walker. There was a long history of suspicion between UT Austin and many of the neighborhood groups in East Austin. This was based on fears about the university expanding into East Austin neighborhoods and displacing many of the area's economically disadvantaged residents. There had been several previous episodes in which the university had purchased land quietly—some neighbors thought surreptitiously— in a manner that might have a negative effect on these neighborhoods. It was crucial, therefore, that there be excellent communication between the university and neighborhood groups for the UT development on the Mueller property to be successful.

Walker had been hired as the Director of the Central Texas Sustainability Indicators Project. From 2001 to 2002, he served as President of the Austin Neighborhoods Council and continued to coordinate many of the activities of neighborhood groups with the City of Austin and outside agencies. He graduated from UT Austin in 1998. He was centrally involved in neighborhood issues, including the redevelopment of the Mueller airport, and served as Chair of the Community and Regional Planning development committee. He regularly briefed the City Council on neighborhood views in East Austin. A crucial part of the communications was to receive an absolute commitment from the university that it would seek no more than twenty-five acres of the Mueller property for the development of a medical school. When the university agreed to restrict itself to fifteen acres, no other formal action was taken on this request. These informal meetings led to a public meeting on January 9, 2005, at the United Way for Greater Austin offices. The Coalition, which included Walker and a number of other community leaders, met with Shine and President Stobo about potential developments (President Stobo attended several of these informal community meetings).

At a community meeting on June 8, 2005, Dr. Stobo reiterated his commitment to an open-door approach to communications between UT Medical Branch and the community. He outlined the variety of UT Medical Branch activities in Austin. He also suggested the development of a community clinic for low-income families in proximity to the medical school site. Shine described the vision for the medical school in greater detail, including the construction of a research institute devoted to pediatrics that would be located near the developing Dell Children's Hospital. Representatives of community groups were particularly interested in traffic patterns and a desire to ensure that 51st Street, which abuts the Mueller property, would be kept open for a potential rail line. The overall project update and acquisition procedures were outlined by Greg Weaver, Managing Director and President of Catellus, the developer for the former Mueller airport site project. Shine and Stobo provided an update on the university's view of the project, including the potential economic impact and philanthropic donors, as well as the community services that would be provided. Local architects Girard Kinney and David Andrews presented detailed information about the architectural plans for the development. The group then moved to a series of tables at which community members met with representatives of the university and the planners. Representatives from the City of Austin participated in the discussion of various topics. The tables considered community services, additional land needs and locations, traffic impact, employment numbers, and salary ranges, as well as economic impact, affordable housing, and other non–UT related Mueller questions. The general tenor of the meeting was positive. Media coverage (InFact News) quoted Jim Walker, Chair of the Mueller Municipal Plan Advisory Committee, as saying that "he was pleased with the progress of talks with UT System. The University has come back with answers that the neighbors are raising about the health science complex." One of the major concerns was the desire of the neighborhood to replace the 111 units of housing that would be lost by converting residential space to nonresidential use in order to support the medical programs.

The Mueller Neighborhoods Coalition met almost monthly throughout 2005 and 2006 to consider development plans for the Mueller site. Shine and other representatives of the UT System, including John De La Garza, the UT System Vice Chancellor for Community Relations, attended almost all of these meetings. The Coalition was particularly interested in how Catellus had developed an academic campus for the University of California, San Francisco, at the Mission Bay location. Greg Weaver provided a summary of these developments. The members of the Robert Mueller Municipal Airport Plan Implementation Advisory Commission are shown in appendix 7.

Discussions with community groups about the Mueller site were briefly negatively impacted by another land issue involving UT Austin. The university was in the process of building a large conference center and hotel and sought to acquire an adjacent property that housed a popular local restaurant called Players. The university proposed to use the land occupied by Players for the construction of a 1,000-space parking garage in conjunction with the new hotel and conference center. The owners of Players, who were UT graduates themselves, were unreceptive to the university's attempts to purchase the property at appraised values. In November 2004, the Board of Regents approved using eminent domain to acquire the property. The owners of Players strongly resisted these attempts and demanded a much larger amount of money to sell their restaurant and land. They hired an attorney and engaged a number of politicians to oppose the university. After the flurry of activity over the Players incident, the university proceeded with the construction of the conference center and hotel without further attempts to acquire the restaurant. (UT Austin acquired the Players property much later, in 2013, at a price close to that originally demanded by the owners, through a combination of university and foundation funding that allowed the payment of substantially more than the appraised value.) To the community representatives, this 2004 activity appeared to be a one-sided power play by the university to annex land by eminent domain. It also reactivated painful history from over a decade before, when UT Austin had begun to accumulate land east of I-35, which could substantially displace poor individuals, particularly African Americans, from their homes. The manner in which these acquisitions took place infuriated community members and created significant distrust, requiring a prolonged period of discussion, communication, and negotiation. For a period of time, the Players incident unsettled the neighborhood associations, but through much effort and conversation, trust was reestablished with the UT Medical Branch and UT System over a number of months.

The UT System and UTMB addressed other issues during conversations about the Mueller development, such as concerns about biocontainment (hazardous material) research. This concern was easily addressed because no such hazardous material–related research would take place at the Mueller site. It was noted that any vivarium would use only small animals, e.g., mice, rats, rabbits, in research. A question was raised about the role of the UT Medical Branch in providing care for prisoners in the Texas correctional system. This was identified as irrelevant to the Mueller development.

Weaver, the Catellus manager of the Mueller Community Development, actively supported opportunities to locate medical facilities at the Mueller site and was specifically supportive of the creation of a pediatric research institute, which would become the Dell Pediatric Research Institute.

THE UT MEDICAL BRANCH CONNECTION

Periodically, UTMB constituents questioned whether UTMB was moving to Austin. In an editorial by Heber Taylor in the *Galveston Daily News* on July 24, 2005, he emphasized that UTMB had been a leader in Texas medicine and that a medical school was "going to be built in Austin regardless of whether the people in Galveston think that's a good idea."[8] Taylor emphasized that Dr. Jack Stobo, the President of the UT Medical Branch, "has been unequivocal about his vision for the campus in Austin. It will be built only if new private monies come from the Austin community in the amount of approximately $100 million. The students who attend will be new. The faculty will be new faculty. In every question, when asked about whether the commitment to a campus in Austin would dilute the commitment to Galveston, the answer was no."[9] Taylor concluded that if there were to become a medical school in Austin, it (UTMB) should lead this new venture because it can. "It's good at working with other institutions, it already trains medical students through cooperative programs in Austin, it has agreements with hospitals and physician groups in Austin and has a long history of reaching out to meet needs in other parts of the State."[10] Taylor went on to say, "People in Galveston and Galveston County, rather than worrying about being abandoned, should worry about missing an opportunity. It's an opportunity for a homegrown institution to get bigger and stronger. We're all better served by that."[11]

On November 21, 2005, the Seton Healthcare Family and the UT Medical Branch announced a thirty-year agreement to double the number of medical residents who received specialty training in Austin over the next five years (appendices 8 and 9). This development was described by Dr. Thomas Blackwell, UT Medical Branch Senior Associate Dean for Austin Initiatives, as an agreement that "will propel undergraduate and GME in Austin. It changes these programs from being community-based programs to academic university-based programs."[12]

THE DELL DEVELOPMENT

Michael Dell is a global business leader and philanthropist in Austin. While a freshman at UT Austin, he developed a business selling upgrade kits for personal computers. He left the university and created a company—later to become Dell Technologies—based on direct sales of personal computers from the manufacturer to the user. In 1999, Mi-

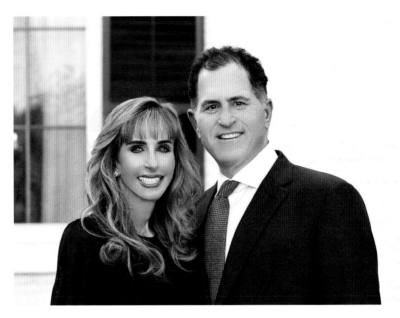

Michael and Susan Dell

chael and Susan Dell created their family foundation, the Michael & Susan Dell Foundation, with the mission of transforming the lives of children living in urban poverty through improved education, health, and family economic stability. The foundation has been instrumental in driving the improvement of childhood health and family health in Austin, with over $200 million in support of medical research, education, hospital capacity, and clinical services.

Janet Mountain was an executive at Dell Inc., where she led several business units and served as Vice President and General Manager. She graduated from UT Austin with a bachelor's in business administration and later received a master's in business administration from Harvard Business School. In early 2003, Susan and Michael Dell asked her to help lead the foundation. She became an important adviser to the Dells and built the foundation team from the ground up. She played a critical role in the creation of the DPRI and the support and naming of the new medical school at UT Austin.

Following the advice of Pete Winstead, Randa Safady contacted

Mountain to discuss the potential for a medical school. This led to an exchange of information and a series of meetings with Mountain. Shine approached Stobo with the concept of a pediatric research institute as the first step in developing the academic medical center in Austin. Stobo was enthusiastic about the idea, and the two met with Mountain and her team. Subsequent discussions included the development of a proposal for the research institute, along with a more complete vision for the establishment of the medical school, both of which were later shared with Susan and Michael Dell. In the proposals, Shine collected data to demonstrate the amount of research funding utilized by UT and other medical schools across the country. The data demonstrated that if UT Medical Branch and UT Austin were a single campus, they would rank eighth in the United States for research funding in 2003. Initial meetings stressed the general concept of a medical school and its potential contribution to UT Austin and the Greater Austin area, as well as the state and national impact. Discussions regarding the loca-

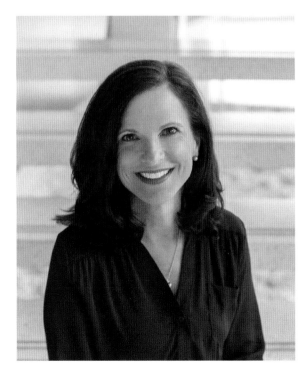

Janet Mountain

tion of a medical school on the Mueller site had advanced to the point that it was proposed as the location for an initial discussion.

Philip Aldridge, the Assistant Vice Chancellor for Business Affairs at the UT System, prepared a series of financial projections that would be useful in the creation of the UTMB academic health center. This took the form of two distinct financial steps. Stage 1 was focused on the creation of a research building (of 180,000 square feet) on the Mueller site. It was also proposed to have 20,000 square feet of retail space and a 460-space parking garage. The total capital cost was estimated at $118 million. Stage 2 involved two additional research facilities, a classroom auditorium building, a library, offices for faculty and administration, a parking garage with 475 spaces, and a potential VA clinic (VA-funded). The total capital cost was estimated at $407 million. Aldridge projected that the overall operational funding requirements for Stages 1 and 2 would total $1.4 million. It was assumed that a substantial portion of these costs, estimated at $330 million, would come from philanthropy. Aldridge's calculations benefited from information and advice provided by Kevin Hegarty, Chief Financial Officer for UT Austin.

At a meeting on May 9, 2005, with Kendall Pace of the Dell Foundation, Safady and Shine discussed major elements involved in the creation of other top medical schools, and Pace asked for additional information about the top twenty ranked schools. They also discussed the "world-class" attributes of a medical school.

At a meeting between Safady, Aldridge, Shine, Mountain, and Pace on August 31, 2005, the group reviewed the UT Medical Branch proposal for a freestanding medical school campus or a medical school as part of UT Austin. They considered the development of a medical research campus at Mueller as a first step without a commitment to begin the medical school until additional resources were available. Shine was asked for an alternative if the UT Medical Branch option was not acceptable. He indicated that a medical school as part of the UT Austin campus would be the best way to create a world-class program and help UT Austin reach its full potential. Shine reviewed the significant reservations on the campus about taking on major additional financial commitments and reiterated that any debt would be managed by the UT

System rather than UT Austin. Dell Foundation staff asked about reporting relationships, and Shine indicated that should the foundation want to proceed with the UT Austin model, the UT System would have to bring campus representatives to the table. The Dell Foundation staff indicated they would like to promptly bring the process to a conclusion.

Following a meeting in early July 2005, Pace reported on a meeting with the Dells that indicated there was support for the Shine proposal, and discussion began regarding a more formal briefing for the Dells by UT Austin leadership.

In subsequent meetings with staff at the Dell Foundation, Shine outlined his concept of the incremental development of an academic health center, beginning with a pediatric research institute, followed by additional research institutes and academic and/or teaching facilities as funds became available. Dell Foundation staff reported to Safady that the Dells were interested in playing a role in these developments.

President Mountain then scheduled a briefing for Susan and Michael Dell on October 14, 2005, at the offices of the Dell Foundation. Present at the meeting were Susan and Michael Dell, Mountain, Board of Regents Chair James Huffines, Chancellor Mark Yudof, President of UT Austin Larry Faulkner, Shine, Aldridge, and Safady. The meeting was opened by Chair Huffines, speaking to the importance of the initiative and his belief that the Board of Regents would contribute funds to the effort. Chancellor Yudof reiterated the UT System's support and emphasized the strength of the existing UT Health Science Center campuses as participants in the effort. President Faulkner conveyed the interest and support for UT Austin and the sense that a medical presence would make the institution play a more significant role nationally. Shine then gave a PowerPoint presentation describing the intent to create a world-class medical school with innovations in education, research, patient care, technology transfer, and community impact. The presentation described specific synergies between the medical school and the UT Austin campus, as well as the commitment of Seton to medical education and world-class patient care. Shine outlined a plan for developing the medical school in stages. Local political and community support for the medical school was identified. Aldridge was prepared to discuss the financial requirements, which seemed daunting at the time.

On October 27, 2005, Safady consulted with Mountain, who indicated that the Dell Foundation would like to revisit the original plan of an incremental approach beginning with the pediatric research institute (children's health and research). The location of the facility would be on the fifteen-acre tract, which the City of Austin would lease to the UT System for $1 a year for ninety-nine years. Thomas and Florence Mayne, then UT System Executive Director of Real Estate, successfully finalized the lease with the City of Austin. A lease requirement was that construction of a second facility on the land must be initiated no later than 2015. Although this term was not met, the City of Austin agreed not to enforce the requirement in view of the subsequent establishment of a full-fledged medical school.

UT SYSTEM BOARD OF REGENTS RETREAT

At a retreat of the Board of Regents in December 2005, Shine reviewed the status of a possible academic health center for Austin. At that time, Shine emphasized the creation of a medical research institute. On January 16, 2006, Dr. Mary Ann Rankin, Dean of the College of Natural Sciences at UT Austin, indicated that she supported the creation of a medical research institute that would probably be focused on child development, nutrition, and general developmental biology, and would have connections to UT Medical Branch and other UT System medical schools, would provide opportunities for clinical programs by the new Dell Children's Hospital, and would be funded initially with private donations of $100 million to $110 million and, later, by indirect cost return from research grants. It would be part of UT Austin, reporting to the Provost and President. Rankin went on to say, "Both Bill Powers [President-designate] and I were asked to comment on whether or not this would be welcomed at UT Austin, and we both said it would be, with the caveat, that adequate funding needed to be available so as not to drain funds away from other essential programs." She noted that a fairly lengthy discussion ensued with regard to the possibilities of a medical school and its location, but indicated that "no solution was reached except to explore further the possibility of private funding for the medical institution."[13]

UT SYSTEM BOARD OF REGENTS PROGRESS REPORT

In August 2004, Shine had presented a set of principles (appendix 5) to the Board of Regents to guide the creation of an Austin academic health center that might eventually lead to a medical school. In January 2006, Chair Huffines requested that Shine provide an update to the Board of Regents on the development of the center. On January 12, 2006, Shine made a PowerPoint presentation (appendices 10 and 11) in which he reiterated the principles that would guide the development of such a center. These included the requirement that it be of the highest quality, be approached incrementally with adequate funding at each step, require considerable private support, be proximate to UT Austin (including the potential use of the Mueller site), and create a partnership between UT Austin and other UT Health Science centers. Shine emphasized that such a center could include medical education, research, nursing and pharmacy education, a regional public health campus, and substantial healthcare programs provided in collaboration with community hospitals. Shine reported that Catellus was supportive of the City of Austin's desire to provide fifteen acres as part of a long-term lease to support the beginnings of an academic health center. In addition, Shine indicated that with City Council approval, UT Austin might purchase an additional adjacent ten acres. Such a site could accommodate four research buildings, educational buildings, and a potential VA clinic, and would be proximate to Dell Children's Hospital. Shine reported on continuing interactions with neighborhood organizations that were comfortable with the design features developed for such a site, provided there was assurance UT Austin would not expand beyond twenty-five acres. He also indicated that there might be a retail component to the buildings and potential for a small children's museum dedicated to health.

Shine's presentation included a review of UT Medical Branch clinical programs in Austin. These included a women's hospital, the OB/ GYN residency program, the signing of a 2005 UT Medical Branch/Seton/UT System affiliation agreement, the presence of approximately 120 UT Medical Branch medical students annually in Austin, and the development of an MD/PhD program between the UT Medical Branch and UT Austin. He also noted efforts to create an imaging center, which would be a joint venture of the UT Medical Branch, the VA, and UT Austin. There was increased interest by supportive community clinics. There was a specific discussion of the potential for biomedical research institutes with strong components of translational research to bring basic science to the bedside. This included a children's health research institute (appendix 12), which would include developmental biology, genetics, and nutrition, as discussed with Dean Rankin. Additionally, an institute for nursing science and/or an institute for heart disease or cancer were being considered. Shine indicated that there was strong community support for this effort, which was broad-based and would contribute significantly to economic development in Central Texas and meet community health needs. He concluded with a series of next steps, which included the continuation of clinical/educational programs, ongoing efforts to enhance UT Austin collaborations with health campuses, and the pursuit of philanthropic opportunities focused upon a biomedical research institution, especially in children's health research. Although the Board of Regents took no formal action on the presentation, the general tone of the discussion indicated continued support along the lines that Shine articulated. This was another critical milestone as the Board of Regents became more comfortable with the development of medical/health programs in Austin.

REGENTS' MEETING AFTERMATH

On February 13, 2006, James Huffines reported to Shine and Safady that the Mayor of Austin, Will Wynn, had called about a number of items and explained that he was aware of quite a bit of pushback from Austin community leaders who thought the Mueller site was too small for the development of a medical school. The Mayor made it perfectly clear that he would take charge and help them work out the problem. Huffines thanked him for his offer and explained that UT teams were exploring all options and would get back to him. He also told Wynn that UT was open to his help if it was determined further adjustments were needed on the proposed site.

On the same day, Mark Yudof indicated that he had spoken with Pete Winstead about the location of the pediatric institute. Yudof quoted Winstead as saying that the Dell Children's Hospital was critical for the Dells—a deal breaker if you went elsewhere. Safady responded by saying she thought we needed to consider with the Dells the important bedside benefits that we could get from the DPRI in close proximity to the Dell's Children's Hospital on the Mueller site, and other important phase 2 parts of the academic health center that may fit on 25 acres. But that further expansion, over a number of years, might lend itself to other sites if opportunities don't present themselves at the Mueller site. During this time, preliminary discussions occurred with Richard Eiason, who was Vice President for Development on the UT Austin campus. He indicated great enthusiasm for the creation of a medical program and medical facilities and believed that fundraising could be very successful for such a project. Safady continued her vigorous activity in supporting the Children's Research Project. She took Zeynep Young, a key staff person at the Dell Foundation, on a tour of the Mueller site. Safady reported that "she was sold on it as are the Dells. So, Pete's [Winstead] assessment is quite accurate." Winstead, who also worked with Catellus to obtain the opportunity for the creation of the Mueller community plan, indicated that he thought the relationships between Shine, President Stobo of the UT Medical Branch, and John De La Garza of the UT System staff, among others, had led to improved relationships with the neighborhood development committee and that "if we can continue the very positive relationship with Jim Walker and his group, they will only be even more supportive of us over time."

The time with the neighborhood development committees was well spent. On April 25, 2006, Safady observed that what seemed to work particularly well with the Mueller group was outreach efforts undertaken by Shine and Stobo. They had many meetings in the Mueller neighborhood environment. Every time the group members posed a question to which they didn't have an answer on the spot, Stobo would come back with an answer later. The Mueller folks felt like they had equity in the project. The neighbors felt like the project was as proposed and was not a fait accompli: comments mattered.

As plans for the DPRI developed, the reporting relationships at UT Austin were examined. Initially, it was thought that the DPRI might report to the Provost as an independent research unit; however, Dean Mary Ann Rankin recommended that the Director of the DPRI report to the Dean of Natural Sciences and through that Dean to the Provost. She proposed an oversight committee to collaborate with the Dean of Natural Sciences and oversee the direction of the DPRI; she also proposed that there be liaison committees between DPRI, the UT Medical Branch, and the general faculty of UT Austin. Ultimately, the DPRI reported to the Dean of Natural Sciences. With the establishment of the Dell Medical School, the DPRI reported to the Dean of the School of Medicine, who then delegated its management to the Chair of Pediatrics.

THE DELL FOUNDATION FOLLOW-UP

After UT System leadership met with Susan and Michael Dell, Janet Mountain advised that the Dells wanted to determine if there were other community leaders with a shared interest in starting a new medical school. They were concerned that they not be seen as "going it alone." Shine, Thomas, and Safady had a number of conversations with community leaders and philanthropists with regard to the potential for a medical school. These conversations were kept very preliminary and private. However, with the support of Chair Huffines and Chancellor Yudof, two dinners were organized at the Chancellor's residence (Bauer House), at which the Chancellor, Chair, and Shine presented a brief overview of the medical school project. These relatively small dinners included fifteen to twenty community leaders who had expressed an interest in the new medical school. During this time, Faulkner stepped down as President of UT Austin, and after a national search, William "Bill" Powers Jr. was selected as President-designate. Powers was among those who participated in these dinners.

The general tenor of the discussions was in support of the vision. The most serious concern, raised by several participants, was the relatively small size of the Mueller tract. Recommendations were made that larger tracts of land, which might grow to a very substantial size, be examined for the location of a medical school. Although no specific attribution was made to Susan and Michael Dell as potential donors, those in the room strongly suspected that the Dells would play an important philanthropic role in the new medical school. In the aftermath of these dinners, several participants indicated that they would strongly consider making donations in support of a new medical school.

DPRI FUNDING

In conversations between Shine, Safady, and the staff of the Dell Foundation during the fall of 2005, a range of philanthropic gifts was discussed that might fund the construction of a pediatric research institute. The conversation began to focus on a $50 million gift, given over ten years, that would be matched by other philanthropic contributions. However, shortly before the foundation made its final decision, two other considerations arose. President Faulkner wrote the Dell Foundation to request a $10 million gift for a new computer science building. UT Austin had not yet placed the building on the Capital Improvement Plan for the Board of Regents, and UT leadership knew that conversations on the pediatric research institute were well down the line. Many observers thought the Dells would still support the computer science building without reducing their $50 million gift for the DPRI.

The staff of the Dell Foundation asked Shine his thoughts about also supporting a project in childhood obesity. Shine suggested they consider the CATCH school health program, conducted by Drs. Deanna Hoelscher and Steven Kelder, faculty of the Austin regional campus of the School of Public Health at UTHSC-Houston. The final gift proposal from the Dell Foundation became $38 million for the DPRI, $10 million for the computer science building, and $2 million for the childhood obesity program.

Most importantly, the Dell Foundation stipulated that the DPRI be part of UT Austin and not operated by the UT Medical Branch, as was originally proposed. As a consequence of this proposal, Chancellor Yudof, Chair Huffines, Shine, and Safady met with Bill Powers, the new President of UT Austin. The group reviewed the Dell Foundation proposal with Powers and asked whether he would accept the money on behalf of UT Austin with all of the conditions, including the construction of a $95 million facility (DPRI), recruitment of a Director, and a commitment to raise an equal amount of money (i.e., $38 million) to match the Dell Foundation gift. The Dells had also stipulated that the building be completed within 36 months in order to make regular payments on the commitment. President Powers agreed, and the Dell Foundation was notified that the Chancellor would recommend to the Board of Regents that they accept the gift on the foundation's terms. The change in sponsorship of the Dell Pediatric Research Institute (DPRI) from UTMB to UT Austin would have a profound impact on the subsequent events in the development of an Austin medical school and on the role of UTMB in Austin.

The Board of Regents approved the Dell Foundation gift and associated naming on May 10, 2006. The Dells publicly announced the gift on May 15, 2006. The Board of Regents formally approved the construction of the DPRI on June 20, 2006, with $38 million from the Dell Foundation, $38 million from other gifts, and $21 million from UT System Revenue Finance System bond proceeds, for a total of $97 million (appendix 13).

The conditions of the gift immediately altered the relationship of UTMB with Austin. President Stobo had traveled frequently to Austin to meet with neighborhood groups and representatives of the Dell Foundation to advance the plan for the research institute. As a consequence of the decision to move the project to UT Austin, President Stobo and UTMB were forced to begin a serious reassessment of their future activities and commitments in Austin.

UT Austin promptly constituted a committee to plan the new DPRI facility, which resulted in a state-of-the-art, 149,653-square-foot building that contained a small-animal vivarium as well as wet labs and dry labs. Construction of the DPRI began on November 6, 2006, and was on schedule for completion six to eight months prior to the three-year deadline required by the Dell Foundation. Unfortunately, completion was delayed when a steam pipe ruptured and a substantial release of hot water and steam resulted in extensive damage to the new building. Ultimately, the contractor repaired the building and bore the principal cost of the accident; however, the incident delayed the opening of the DPRI for eighteen months. The state-of-the-art research facility opened on October 28, 2010 (appendix 14).

There was considerable discomfort with the DPRI on the UT Austin campus. It was initially considered by some in leadership as an unfunded mandate imposed on the campus by the UT System. UT Austin leadership were concerned about the sufficiency and availability of recurring operating funds for the DPRI. There was also concern that philanthropic efforts in support of the facility would detract from other campus priorities and philanthropy, and no serious effort was made by the campus to raise the required matching funds for the building. As a consequence, Safady and Chair Huffines approached the Dell Foundation to determine whether endowment funds managed by the Board of Regents might be used to match their gift. In addition, the Board of Regents would provide additional funding for the construction of the DPRI. The Dell Foundation agreed to this approach, and the Board of Regents designated funds for this purpose on November 8–9, 2007.

There was some concern that the facility, located approximately two miles from the main campus, was too far for faculty to travel, despite its immediate proximity to Dell Children's Hospital. The Dells had also contributed $25 million toward the construction of the children's hospital. The original plan called for the recruitment of a director for the DPRI. UT Austin leaders made no serious efforts to recruit a director. One philanthropist for the DPRI committed $1 million to support the director of the DPRI during its construction. He withdrew the gift after no director was subsequently recruited. The Dell Foun-

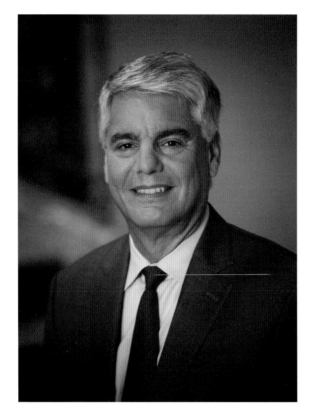

Greg Fenves

dation was concerned and disappointed that no efforts to recruit a director had been made, even though the original budget had included $25 million for a director and additional faculty, had the UT Austin match been raised. UT Austin did little to populate the building with relevant programs until Steve W. Leslie became Executive Vice President and Provost. He worked tirelessly to identify projects that could be effectively located there. Initially, faculty involved in nutrition research were moved to the facility, and, later, a faculty group devoted to cancer research would be located at the DPRI.

In 2015, under the leadership of the new President of UT Austin, Dr. Greg Fenves, interest in recruiting a director for the DPRI and establishing a true pediatric program was reactivated. Subsequently, the

Founding Dean of the Dell Medical School, Dr. Clay Johnston, recruited Dr. Steven Abrams as Chair of Pediatrics. Dr. Abrams saw the DPRI as a great opportunity to conduct research proximate to Dell Children's Hospital, and he actively initiated the recruitment of faculty. He became the first acting Director of the DPRI. Subsequently, he stepped down as Chair of Pediatrics, and a search was launched for his successor. It was unclear whether the new Chair would also be the Director of the DPRI.

THE DPRI ERA: A SUMMARY

The years 2004 through 2009 were a significant transition period for the development of the Dell Medical School. The Board of Regents had been extremely skeptical of a new medical school in Austin. The Shine briefings to the Board of Regents in August 2004 and January 2006 provided a vision for the development of an academic health center in Austin without actually committing to the formal creation of a medical school. The academic health center concept involved the continuation and expansion of undergraduate medical education, principally with students from the UT Medical Branch. It included the continuation and expansion of residency programs with Seton. Seton committed substantial financial support for the residents and faculty who taught them, which provided the basis for a strong clinical enterprise. The creation of the DPRI was a mixed blessing in the short term. It provided an important stake in the ground for a facility dedicated to medical research—in this case, research related to pediatrics. It offered fifteen acres of leased space on the Mueller site that could be further developed if the land was not available on the central UT Austin campus. It started the UT System's concept of an academic health center in a demonstrable and meaningful way. It involved Susan and Michael Dell in direct conversations about the potential for a medical school arising out of the academic health center.[14]

Although a state-of-the-art facility (DPRI) was built for UT Austin, its population and programming were not initially successful. While enthusiastically supported by the leadership of the UT Medical Branch, UT Austin leadership did not initially commit resources. In the absence of active fundraising, the Board of Regents was required to provide the residual funding for the facility. While the DPRI housed some meaningful research, on subjects such as nutrition and cancer, no institute was created or a director recruited. This displeased the Dell Foundation leadership. When the Dells offered $50 million as a naming opportunity for the new UT Austin medical school in 2013, Powers publicly acknowledged that the DPRI had been an important step in the creation of the Dell Medical School.

In the aftermath of the pivotal decision by the Dell Foundation to require that the DPRI be operated by UT Austin, it was clear that further financial support from the Dell Foundation would not be predicated upon collaboration with the UT Medical Branch. Instead, it was apparent that the Dell Foundation would be much more sympathetic to a partnership between UT Austin and UT Southwestern.

This transition period from 2004 to 2009 saw the movement of residency programs from UT Medical Branch sponsorship to UT Southwestern sponsorship. This transition led to early successful foundational planning for a medical school going beyond the concept of an academic health center; with the transfer of the DPRI to UT Austin, the UT Medical Branch significantly reduced its interest in a regional health center in Central Texas and accelerated its planning for expansion north of Galveston Island to areas south of Houston. The UT Medical Branch built important new facilities and programs in that area and relied, to a decreasing extent, on the development of programs in Austin.

This era was also one of activity by the CTI, which contributed to the development and expansion of medical education and research in Austin by virtue of the interactions between its members. Of particular importance was the involvement of Steve Leslie, who would go on to become Executive Vice President and Provost of UT Austin. His background as Dean of the College of Pharmacy provided important insight into healthcare. His understanding of the value of a medical school guided his conversations with UT Southwestern and allowed him to further think about a medical school. Led by Regent Huffines and, later, Chair of the Board of Regents Scott Caven, the UT System began serious planning for a medical school in Austin. Although the UT System and the community were enthusiastically engaged in conversations about creating the new school, few understood the magnitude of the economic downturn that was to impact the nation and Central Texas and put all planning activities on hold.

CHAPTER 5

THE PACE QUICKENS— THEN THE RECESSION

The decision by the Dell Foundation to direct its gift for the DPRI to UT Austin rather than the UTMB dramatically changed the landscape for academic medicine in Austin. It became clear to Stobo and his colleagues that major philanthropic support for the development of UT Medical Branch programs in Austin would be limited, despite broad-based support from its medical school alumni in Austin. Stobo concluded that it would take a significant effort for the UT Medical Branch to establish a clinical presence in the Austin metropolitan area. Stobo continued to support an affiliation of the UT Medical Branch with residency programs at Brackenridge Hospital, but understood the necessity of focusing on the expansion of clinical activities for the UT Medical Branch on Galveston Island, and especially on the mainland near Houston.

FROM UT MEDICAL BRANCH TO UT SOUTHWESTERN

The Board of Regents named David L. Callender, MD, MBA, FACS, as President of the UT Medical Branch in 2007. He succeeded Jack Stobo, who stepped down as President after ten years of able leadership, which included strong support for medical education programs in Austin. After an initial evaluation, Callender concluded that the future of the UT Medical Branch lay in developing programs in the Victory Lakes and Clear Lake areas, between the UT Medical Branch and Houston. He indicated to Shine that he would be open to transferring the UTMB sponsorship of residency programs in Austin to another UT institution. He planned for UTMB medical students to continue their rotations in Austin, with the expansion of clinical programs at UT Medical Branch eventually allowing for adequate training opportunities for medical student and residency programs in or near Galveston.

HURRICANE HISTORY

Hurricanes have played a remarkable role in the development of medical education and medical schools in the University of Texas System. The 1900 hurricane that decimated Galveston Island destroyed almost the entire UTMB campus, with the exception of "Old Red." However, up to the time of the hurricane, financial support and leadership for the medical school at Galveston from the UT Regents had been minimal. Impressed by the dedication and efforts of students and faculty on the Island during and after the hurricane, the Regents dramatically increased financial resources, as noted previously in this report. Subsequently, UTMB played a substantial role in medical education, patient care, and research for the University of Texas System and the state.

In 2005, Hurricane Katrina struck the southern coast of Texas and Louisiana. Louisiana bore the brunt of this storm. However, in preparation for dealing with the storm, the University of Texas Medical Branch, under the leadership of President Jack Stobo, executed a plan to evacuate essentially all of its patients from the hospital on the island to the mainland. The relationship between UTMB and the Seton Healthcare Family was crucial to the success of these efforts, particularly for infants who were in the neonatal intensive care unit. At the request of UTMB, Seton provided enough beds and staff to care for nineteen infants. Working together substantially enhanced the relationship between the two institutions and demonstrated the extraordinary benefits that arose from such relationships.

In 2008, Hurricane Ike struck Galveston Island, and patients were evacuated to the mainland expeditiously and without complications. Again, the Seton Healthcare Family assisted with the care of UTMB patients, though not to the extent of what had occurred after Hurricane Katrina. An extended rebuilding program was required at UT Medical Branch that ultimately cost in excess of $1.2 billion. Led by Dr. David Callender, the campus recovered from the impact of the hurricane over several years, but it also began a much more extensive planning process in regard to its future. Callender and his colleagues determined that the area of the mainland north of the island and approximately halfway to the city of Houston was the appropriate area for the medical branch to develop new programs. As a result, it indicated a desire to withdraw from the residency programs in Austin. The previous decision to affiliate the DPRI with UT Austin had raised the question of the future of UTMB's presence in Central Texas, but Hurricane Ike and the subsequent planning on the campus forced the decision to withdraw.

UT SOUTHWESTERN–SETON COLLABORATION

After Callender's decision, Shine approached President Kern Wildenthal about the potential for UT Southwestern to sponsor the residency programs at Seton in Austin, prior to the development of a new medical school. Wildenthal was supportive, and negotiations began between UT Southwestern and Seton regarding the transfer of sponsorship of these Austin-based residency programs from UTMB to UT Southwestern.

Seton provided substantial funding for residency programs over the years and proposed continuing to make substantial investments in the programs. For that reason, Seton felt it had a right to control any clinical programs carried out in conjunction with UT Southwestern and that UT Southwestern and other institutions of the UT System should not be allowed to create programs using the University of Texas name without the express permission of Seton. Initially, this was to include research programs; however, the UT System was adamant that there be no limitations on research conducted by any of its faculty at any of its institutions. It was agreed that clinical research conducted in Seton facilities would have to follow Catholic Ethical and Religious Directives. It was also agreed that research at other UT institutions would not be translated directly into a clinical program in Central Texas using the University of Texas name with a Seton competitor. However, all research attributed to the University of Texas was permitted.

After protracted negotiations between UT representatives (Shine, Thomas, Cox, and Barry Burgdorf) and Seton representatives, on November 3, 2009, UT Southwestern and the Seton Healthcare Family entered into an agreement where UT Southwestern assumed sponsorship of the prior UTMB residency programs at Seton. The goal was to increase the number of residencies from approximately 160 positions to significantly more, perhaps 250 positions, within a few years. The UT Medical Branch would continue to send medical students to Austin for clinical rotations in Seton facilities.

The Seton–UT Southwestern agreement included a provision to establish a clinical research group with up to twenty researchers. The creation of this research group at Seton was important to expand clinical research programs in Austin.

Although Shine emphasized that the establishment of a medical school in Austin was the decision of the Board of Regents, it was clear that the Chair of the Board, James Huffines, supported its creation.

Consequently, UT Austin Provost Steve Leslie concluded that working with the leadership of UT Southwestern would be valuable in planning for a medical school. Wildenthal agreed to work with UT Austin's leadership on the potential medical school and assembled a team to articulate a plan. Dr. Cox, a distinguished obstetrician/gynecologist (OB/GYN), moved from Dallas to Austin as UT Southwestern Regional Dean to oversee and grow the residency programs. She would later play a key role in the establishment of the Dell Medical School.

A Seton–UT Southwestern affiliation oversight committee was

constituted and contained equal numbers of representatives of UT Southwestern and Seton, with one of the UT Southwestern chairs occupied by a representative of the UT System, Vice Chancellor Thomas, to approve all major business, operational, and strategic decisions of the partners. It was also explicitly agreed that residents in obstetrics and gynecology would have opportunities to receive training at institutions that were not subject to the Catholic Ethical and Religious Directives in reproductive care. Subsequently, the agreement went smoothly, although some concerns developed when St. David's HealthCare System became the sponsor of UT Austin's athletic programs. However, the sponsorship involved healthcare delivery to only athletes and faculty in the sports programs and did not involve programs for the general campus community or the public.

St. David's Medical Center later approached President Daniel Podolsky, of UT Southwestern, to encourage a relationship between St. David's and UT Southwestern. Podolsky indicated that he was committed to programs at Seton, and that he would continue to support and develop those programs.

SUE COX, MD, BECOMES REGIONAL DEAN

Sue Cox, MD, played a pivotal role in the development of residency programs in Austin, as well as the establishment of the Dell Medical School. Dr. Cox graduated from Baylor College of Medicine and completed her training in obstetrics and gynecology, including a fellowship in maternal and fetal medicine. After two years as Chief of Obstetrics at the University of Kentucky, she joined the faculty of UT Southwestern as medical director of the high-risk pregnancy unit and clerkship director in obstetrics and gynecology. In subsequent years she expanded her responsibilities to include fellowship supervision, and by 2006 she was Dean for all undergraduate and graduate medical education (GME). During this time, she played a key role in the development of objectives for the medical undergraduate curriculum as part of the Liaison Committee on Medical Education (LCME) accreditation process

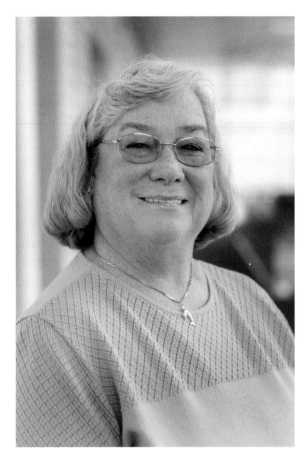

Sue Cox

at UT Southwestern. When UT Southwestern became the principal sponsor for GME for Seton, Dr. Cox oversaw the residency programs. She committed to Austin, beginning in October 2009. She moved to Austin as the Regional Dean on July 1, 2011. Immediately thereafter, she interacted with Senator Watson about his plans to support the creation of a medical school in Austin. Provost Leslie then asked Dr. Cox to become the planning Dean for the new medical school.

In January 2013, after the passage of Central Health Proposition 1 to fund the medical school, Dr. Cox and Dr. Robert Messing, under Provost Leslie's direction, led a steering committee to oversee the development and accreditation of the medical school (appendix 15). Dr. Cox created a task force involving thirteen of the sixteen colleges on the campus, and over 250 people were involved in putting together the medical school curriculum. The vision for the school was articulated (appendix 16). It is remarkably similar to that which the school ultimately achieved. During this time, residents recruited into UT Southwestern–sponsored residency programs at Seton achieved significantly higher United States Medical Licensing Examination scores and greater success in licensure exams than previous residents. UT Southwestern and Seton created additional residency programs, and Dr. Cox played a critical role in negotiating venues in which OB/GYN residents could receive educational experiences beyond those permitted by Catholic Ethical and Religious Directives within Seton facilities. These included rotations at St. David's Hospital, Planned Parenthood clinics, and elsewhere. She also initiated interactions with other health professional schools, particularly nursing, pharmacy, and social work, to create interprofessional education programs.

CENTRAL HEALTH: THE KEY TO A SOLUTION

Central Health was a key participant in the creation of the Dell Medical School. In 2004, with strong support from Kirk Watson and community leader Clarke Heidrick, the voters of Travis County founded Central Health to provide indigent Travis County residents access to healthcare. In addition to providing high-quality, cost-effective care, Central Health was charged with eliminating health disparities and strengthening the safety-net healthcare delivery system. Central Health is governed by a nine-member-appointed Board of Managers. The Austin City Council and Travis County Commissioners Court each appoint four members and jointly appoint a ninth member. Board Members serve four-year terms. Central Health has the authority to authorize and collect ad valorem taxes in support of its mission. In 2009 Senator Watson sponsored legislation that allowed the hospital district to raise the tax rate greater than that currently authorized by Travis County voters. A crucial step in forming the Dell Medical School was a vote in November 2012 to increase the tax rate for the hospital district by $0.05 per $100 assessed value (Proposition 1). This not only increased tax collections for the hospital district but also, under a Medicaid 1115 Waiver, allowed for substantial increases in federal matching funds. Further discussion of this election and the Medicaid Waiver will follow.

During the time that the Chamber of Commerce and community leaders supported the creation of the medical school in Austin, members of the Board of Managers and executive leadership of Central Health also demonstrated a substantial interest in a new medical school. In 2005, Central Health assumed the ownership of Brackenridge Hospital, which Seton continued to manage and operate under contract. Seton also operated the ambulatory clinics and supported a health plan to provide care for medically indigent patients, known as the Medical Access Plan (MAP).

On March 23, 2009, Carole Keeton Strayhorn, then a candidate for Mayor of Austin, appeared at the University Medical Center Brackenridge and made a strong plea for the creation of a medical school in Austin. She was vigorously supported by Dr. William Cunningham, former Chancellor of the UT System and former President of UT Austin; Dr. Charles Mullins, Professor Emeritus at UT Southwestern and former UT System Executive Vice Chancellor for Health Affairs; and industry leaders who formally endorsed former Mayor Strayhorn's candidacy for reelection particularly because of her position on a new medical school. Although Strayhorn did not win the election, her active support of the medical school increased interest in the project across the Austin community.

THE MEDICAL PLAN DEVELOPS

In 2007, President Bill Powers appointed Steve Leslie, then Dean of the College of Pharmacy, to the position of Executive Vice President and Provost of UT Austin. Leslie had a doctorate in pharmacology and toxicology and had previously conducted research that included alcohol's effects on the brain. During Summit 2007, a meeting Leslie helped organize to address medication safety, he became convinced that Austin would benefit from a medical school. As previously noted, he became an original member of the CTI, which had been working on expanding medical education and research programs in Central Texas. With the Board of Regents becoming increasingly receptive to the possibility of a medical school in Austin, Leslie sought to explore plans for its development. It was also clear from discussions with the Dell Foundation that the Dells were very supportive of the relationship between the UT Austin campus and UT Southwestern.

In early 2008, Wildenthal, responding to a request by Shine, agreed to work with Provost Leslie and the UT System to explore the financial feasibility of starting a modest-sized, high-quality, research-oriented medical school in Austin. Wildenthal believed that at some time in the future a major research university such as UT Austin would have a medical school. He thought that collaboration between UT Southwestern and UT Austin to create a medical school could be mutually beneficial and might further enhance, rather than diminish, the status of UT Southwestern and its reputation. Leslie established a small group to work on a feasibility plan for such a medical school. It included Wildenthal, Chief Financial Officer of UT Southwestern John Roan, the newly appointed Dean of the College of Pharmacy at UT Austin M. Lynn Crismon, Dean of the College of Natural Sciences Mary Ann Rankin, Shine, and Thomas. From time to time, Alfred Gilman, the Dean of UT Southwestern Medical School and a Nobel Laureate, along with other staff at UT Southwestern, also contributed to the conversations.

The group detailed assumptions and projections that outlined the creation and start-up of such a school. The assumptions included the creation of a top-tier medical school of a quality comparable to UT Austin. Seton's Brackenridge and Dell Pediatric Hospitals would be the primary teaching hospitals, with other Seton hospitals, and possibly St. David's HealthCare Partnership, providing additional teaching sites. The plan envisioned the eventual creation of a 100-percent full-time faculty at Brackenridge and emphasized that the primary location of the medical school would be as close as possible to Brackenridge and the UT Austin academic campus, with pediatric programs located at the Mueller site near Dell Children's Hospital. The initial class size would be 50, for a total enrollment of 200. Ultimately, there would be 350 residents and fellowship positions and approximately 300 full-time-equivalent faculty members. UT faculty would participate in a typical faculty practice plan, in keeping with other UT schools.

The proposal focused on high-priority interactions between medical school faculty and UT Austin faculty in fields ranging from computer science and chemistry to business and public policy. Wildenthal estimated a total onetime start-up cost, excluding construction costs, of $347.9 million (in 2008 dollars). The plan outlined how the hospitals, philanthropy, the UT System, UT Austin, and Central Health might cover these costs. The planning was very detailed and strongly based on the management experience at UT Southwestern. Some members of the working group thought that the total cost was significantly greater than what was needed to establish a medical school because of the extraordinarily high standards and ambitions of the UT Southwestern participants. However, the draft work paper proved extremely useful in focusing the attention of all participants, especially the leadership at the UT Austin campus, on the possibilities and requirements of creating a medical school.

Shine had been working on another set of financial projections regarding a new medical school that was not as expensive as those detailed in the Wildenthal work paper. Leslie and Shine agreed that a balance between the two approaches would be feasible. Crucial to either plan was the necessity for the availability of local tax dollars from Central Health. Shine approached Senator Watson with this approach, in view of his history and extensive knowledge of and involvement with Central Health and his role as a community leader. A meeting was held with Senator Watson and a number of community leaders at Watson's office in 2008. Shine and Leslie presented the overall strategy and the need for local tax dollars to fund a new medical school. They did not request a specific amount of money at the meeting. Senator Watson generally supported moving forward with a medical school and agreed that approaching Travis County voters was feasible.

In very preliminary discussions, Chair of the Board of Regents Scott Caven and Regent Huffines considered the possibility of a major investment by the Board of Regents in the new medical school. They suggested that $200 million in PUF dollars for construction might become available and $100 million in AUF might be provided for operations of the medical school.

Unfortunately, within a few months of these planning efforts and conversations, the 2008 economic downturn began. This decreased the likelihood of successfully financing a new medical school and of taxpayers approving a tax increase. Shine informed Senator Watson that the UT System would put the project on hold until the economy improved.

The overall economic downturn also dramatically affected the UT endowment. According to Bruce Zimmerman, then President of the University of Texas Investment Management Company (the endowment management company for the UT System and Texas A&M), the downturn caused a 13 percent decline in the value of the endowment, which amounted to approximately $2.3 billion. Funding from the endowment was clearly not feasible at the time.

MEDICAL SCHOOL PUT ON HOLD

In spite of the abrupt termination of activity to create the medical school in the wake of the economic downturn, Shine continued to formulate a bare-bones financial plan that might work to initiate a medical school on a much stricter budget yet also allow for the fulfillment of long-term objectives. It was this financial plan that ultimately became the basis for proceeding with the new school (appendix 17).

Wildenthal concluded twenty-two years as President of UT Southwestern on August 31, 2008, and Dr. Dan Podolsky succeeded him on September 1, 2008. Podolsky had previously served as a Professor at Harvard Medical School and the Chief of Gastroenterology at Massachusetts General Hospital. Podolsky was also the Chief Academic Officer of Partners HealthCare System. Podolsky supported UT Southwestern's sponsorship of residency programs in Austin and became an active participant in discussions about forging a new agreement with Seton. As previously noted, a new affiliation agreement between UT Southwestern and Seton was negotiated during the summer and fall of 2009. In October 2009, the UT Medical Branch transferred sponsorship of its long-standing Austin-based residency programs to UT Southwestern. Seton committed to continue fully funding the residency programs and the faculty to educate the residents. This same faculty also taught medical students from UTMB, who continued to spend time during their third year as clerks at Seton and to participate in fourth-year clerkships. This commitment was a major factor in the ability to start a new medical school.

During the period that Wildenthal, Shine, Thomas, and colleagues were working on plans for the medical school in Austin, and several months prior to the agreement for UT Southwestern sponsorship of residency programs, William T. Solomon, Chair of the Southwestern Medical Foundation, communicated to Chair of the Board of Regents Scott Caven, Vice Chair James Huffines, and Shine great concern about these developments.

On April 29, 2008, Solomon wrote on behalf of twelve of the "strongest pillars of the University of Texas Southwestern Medical Center's philanthropic support base" that they understood their commitment to be "supportive of what the Board of Regents deemed to be in the best interest of the UT System and the State."[1] They indicated an understanding of the rationale on the part of the Austin community "for developing a first-rate medical school."[2] However, the group "expressed serious concern over the current proposal's potential for diverting human and financial resources and leadership focus away from the continued development of UT Southwestern in Dallas at a critical moment in its ascendancy."[3] The group also indicated concern that the involvement could divert time and effort away from the mission at UT Southwestern and that it might also become a substitute for similar collaboration between UT Southwestern and UT Dallas, thereby delaying UT Dallas's attainment of the status wanted for it. The group expressed a "sense that the Dallas philanthropic community could support the launching of a UT Southwestern branch in Austin if UT Southwestern is allowed first to become all that it can be by focusing its available resources entirely on that goal while at the same time leveraging UT Dallas toward Tier 1 status by way of closer collaboration between the two Dallas schools."[4]

Shine responded on behalf of the UT System to assure the philanthropists that there was no intention of diverting significant human or financial resources away from the development at UT Southwestern at this "critical time."[5] The principal short-term commitment was to the establishment of UT Southwestern sponsorship of the residency programs in Austin, which was not unlike their sponsorship of programs in Fort Worth and other communities. It was emphasized that entirely new resources would be required for a medical school in Austin. In a follow-up letter on June 9, 2008, Solomon again asserted the concern of the philanthropists, who were among the most important leaders of the Dallas community, about UT Southwestern's involvement in Austin. It was striking that many of these philanthropists were also strong supporters of UT Austin, in addition to their support for UT Dallas. As events unfolded, UT Southwestern provided excellent sponsorship of their residency programs in Austin, all of which were overseen by Dr. Sue Cox, who was delegated from Dallas full-time to Austin. The chairs of the various departments at UT Southwestern continued to provide oversight for these programs, although a level of anxiety about the long-term future and the time commitments of the faculty at UT Southwestern became problematic. With the establishment of the Dell Medical School, sponsorship of the residency programs was subsequently transferred to Dell Medical School on July 1, 2014.

In order to maintain the momentum toward the creation of an academic health center including the medical school, Shine proposed an additional facility that might be located on the Mueller site. This facility would be the UT System's Center for Health Professionals Education at Austin and would include space for clinical research and rooms for interdisciplinary health education. It would also include a "smart hospital," with state-of-the-art mannequins for interdisciplinary education and training of multi-health professional students, including nursing, public health, pharmacy, health policy, and medical students. This proposal was ultimately encompassed in new buildings for the Dell Medical School.

Additional progress was made in expanding potential medical activities with the recruitment in the summer of 2011 of Robert Messing from the University of California, San Francisco, as previously noted. Messing was a very accomplished neurologist who was a principal investigator at the Ernest Gallo Clinic and Research Center at the University of California, San Francisco. An accomplished researcher and teacher, Messing was the first recruitment to the UT Austin campus around whom a medical school could be envisioned. He ultimately played a role in the negotiation of affiliation agreements between the new medical school and Seton and between the medical school and Central Health. He also worked closely with Sue Cox to obtain the school's initial accreditation.

CHAPTER 6

THE ACTION PLAN

A COHERENT PLAN DEVELOPS

In February 2009, Francisco Cigarroa succeeded Mark Yudof as Chancellor of the UT System. A distinguished transplant surgeon, Cigarroa had previously served as President of UTHSC–San Antonio for ten years. He was considered an outstanding leader and thinker in higher education, including his field of health and healthcare. When Yudof left the Chancellorship at the UT System to become President at the University of California System, the Board of Regents asked Shine to serve as interim Chancellor. He served for nine months with the support of Thomas until Cigarroa became Chancellor. In Shine's conversations with Cigarroa, it became clear that the new Chancellor had an open mind about the possibility of a new medical school in Austin.

In 2011, the Governor appointed three new Regents who, with Chair Gene Powell of San Antonio, expressed great interest in making fundamental changes to the way the UT System, and particularly UT Austin, was managed, was organized, and functioned. They quickly constituted a series of task forces to address these issues. There was a dramatic increase in the amount of data being required by these new Regents, with special attention given to requests by Regent Wallace Hall for extensive information and voluminous documentation from

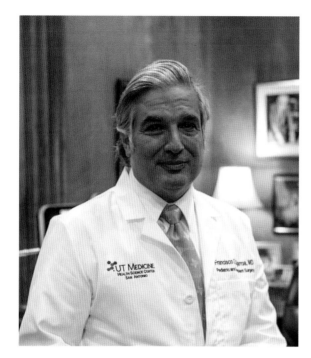

Francisco
Cigarroa

UT Austin. The Board of Regents became polarized, with five Regents espousing traditional concepts of the function of higher education versus four Regents with very different attitudes. Cigarroa was faced with a situation of contention and, in some cases, disruption. In the spring of 2011, he first articulated an overall vision for the future of the UT System's institutions: The Framework for Advancing Excellence Throughout the University of Texas System. Thomas advised Cigarroa on the preparation, substance, and drafting of the Framework. In August 2011, Cigarroa presented the Framework in some detail to the Board of Regents, which they unanimously adopted. The Framework strongly supported enhanced medical education and research in Austin and South Texas. This did not resolve some of the contentious activities of four members of the Board, but it did largely stabilize the Board for the next several years.

Included in that vision was the expansion of educational opportunities in medicine and health in South Texas and Austin. Chair Powell and a number of other Regents had deep roots in South Texas and were very supportive of expanding medical education in the Lower Rio Grande Valley. It became clear that there was an opportunity for parallel developments of medical schools in both locations. This was a major step toward the consideration and development of a medical school in Austin.

Although the previous Chancellor, Yudof, had quietly supported a new medical school in Austin, Cigarroa's statements in the spring and summer of 2011 were the first clear articulation of support by the UT System for the creation of new medical schools in Austin and South Texas.

Legal opinions were sought regarding the authority of the Board of Regents to establish a medical school. Steven Collins, former Executive Director of the Texas Legislative Council and Associate Vice Chancellor and Special Counsel in the Office of Government Relations, researched the issue and reported that existing statutory authority under Texas Education Code §74.201 authorized the Board of Regents to establish and maintain an additional medical school of the university system at any location in the state. However, the Board of Regents must determine that the location of the medical school is in the best interests of the people of the State of Texas, and the doctor of medicine degree must be approved by the Coordinating Board. It was this opinion that led to the Board of Regents' agreement to create and provide funds for a medical school in Austin (appendix 18).

SENATOR KIRK WATSON'S 10 GOALS IN 10 YEARS

The period from late 2009 to early 2011 was one of consolidation of the medical residency programs with the establishment of additional programs under Cox, the Austin Regional Dean for UT Southwestern. As the economy in Central Texas rebounded from the recession and the UT System endowment began to recover significantly, there was renewed interest in the establishment of a medical school. In January 2011, Thomas, who was active in civic affairs in the City of Austin, reported to Shine that conversations were taking place in many influential community organizations, such as AARO, the DAA, and the Chamber of Commerce, that were enthusiastically attempting to support a medical school, often with very different views and concepts about how this might happen. Shine and Thomas concluded that some kind of coordinated effort would be timely in galvanizing community support, and Thomas emphasized the need for a strong champion of a new medical school who was outside the UT family.

In February 2011, Charles Barnett, CEO of Seton, Greg Hartman, and Thomas met in Shine's office to discuss the possibilities. There was agreement that the creation of a community group in the form of a committee of some kind would be timely in bringing together all of the interested parties in support of a medical school. After considering a number of options, the group concluded that the ideal chair for such a committee was Senator Watson. He had been promoting the possibility of a medical school for a decade or more. As a former Mayor and then a successful State Senator, he had gravitas, influence, and broad-based respect in the community. He also had a personal interest in improving health, being a cancer survivor himself.

Hartman agreed to approach Senator Watson about the possibility of leading the effort for a new medical school in Austin, followed by the same request by Shine. The Senator agreed and indicated that he would like to provide leadership for the effort but would be unable to do so until the conclusion of the 2011 Texas legislative session in June 2011. The Governor called a special session of the Texas Legislature that summer, so it was not until September 2011 that Senator Watson was able to devote his time to this endeavor.

Sandy Guzman, Senator Watson's Legislative Director, provided crucial staff support for Watson's efforts to start a new medical school in Austin. She received her undergraduate degree from George Washington University, in Washington, D.C., and worked for a Congressman until she moved to Austin. She worked for the Chamber of Commerce until 2008. During that time, she became aware of UT Medical Branch's medical education and research activities in Austin and the creation of Central Health. In 2005, Senator Watson chaired the Chamber of Commerce and became familiar with Guzman, later hiring her as a member of his staff for the 2009 legislative session. She had attended legislative hearings regarding the rebuilding of UTMB after Hurricane Ike devastated that campus and was familiar with the history of attempts to move the UT Medical Branch medical school to Austin. Her regular legislative duties did not include health, but Senator Watson assigned her to support him with formulating a strategy and approach to starting a new medical school in Austin.

By mid-August of 2011, Guzman and Senator Watson established a list of sixteen action items after conferring regularly with Shine, Thomas, Heidrick, Hartman, and many other community leaders who represented many different constituencies but clearly shared similar interests in areas such as mental health and the potential for a medical school. By mid-September 2011, Watson had pared down the list to ten items.

With support from excellent staff, particularly Guzman and Edna Butts, General Counsel on his staff, Senator Watson created a vision and initiative called 10 Goals in 10 Years. The goals included:

1. Build a medical school
2. Build a modern teaching hospital
3. Establish modern, uniquely Austin health clinics in our neighborhoods
4. Develop laboratories and other facilities for public and private research
5. Launch a new commercialization incubator
6. Make Austin a center for comprehensive cancer care
7. Provide needed psychiatric care and facilities
8. Improve basic infrastructure and create a sense of place
9. Bolster the medical examiner's office
10. Solve the funding puzzle

Watson launched his plan at a major luncheon of the Real Estate Council of Austin on September 20, 2011 (appendix 19). He emphasized that "interested parties resist the temptation to keep waiting, watching, and wishing."[1] He declined to make an estimate of the cost involved in implementing the goals, indicating that it was part of the puzzle to be solved. Senator Watson noted Cigarroa's support of two new medical schools, including one in Austin and another in South Texas. Senator Watson quickly established an organizing committee that included Cigarroa and Shine. UT Southwestern's Greg Fitz, Executive Vice President for Academic Affairs and Provost and Dean of the Medical School, and Dr. Cox were members. Steve Leslie and Bill Powers were also members of the committee. Charles Barnett represented Seton, and David Huffstutler represented St. David's HealthCare Partnership. Central Health was represented by Tom Coopwood and the 2012 Central Health Board Chair, Rosie Mendoza. Additional members were Jeff Garvey of the Austin Community Foundation; Clarke Heidrick, Chair of the Chamber of Commerce; Doug Ulman of the LiveStrong Foundation; Mayor Lee Leffingwell of the City of Austin; and Travis County Judge Sam Biscoe. Senator Watson also added a member from the Travis County Medical Society. There was broad-based support for Senator Watson's effort.

During this time, representatives of St. David's HealthCare System, including Jon Foster and Huffstutler, indicated their support for a medical school but were deeply concerned about the role Seton would play in Senator Watson's 10 Goals in 10 Years. They were adamant that no public money be used for the construction of a new hospital that would compete with St. David's facilities (none was used for this purpose). The opportunity to draw down federal funding through an 1115 Medicaid Waiver made the tax increase much more attractive to accomplishing the 10 Goals.

Ultimately, Senator Watson convened representatives of Central Health and Seton, as well as other knowledgeable individuals, to create the Community Care Collaborative (CCC) as a vehicle through which additional federal funds would flow. Watson then worked closely with the Texas Health and Human Services Commission and the Centers for Medicare and Medicaid Services to accomplish this goal.

In January 2012, a 501(c)(3) was established, titled Healthy ATX, to offer speaker groups, videos, and other mechanisms to educate the public about the benefits of a medical school in Austin. These efforts increasingly focused on the need for Travis County voters to increase property taxes to help fund the medical school. This became part of Central Health Proposition 1. Early polls indicated that a vote on such a proposition had to be done at the time of the presidential election in November 2012 if it were to have a reasonable chance of passage; the larger and broader turnout during a presidential election was much more likely to approve the proposition than during an off-year election.

After the successful Central Health election and establishment of the medical school, Watson encouraged the school to conduct programs at the Austin State Hospital under a new Chair of Psychiatry and to establish neighborhood health clinics. These were important components of the "10 in 10" proposal. The development of an "innovation zone" in Austin continues.

FUNDING THE NEW MEDICAL SCHOOL

Shine had developed a financial plan for a medical school at UT Austin. There was a long-standing agreement that the UT System would not request funds from the Texas Legislature for this purpose. This was particularly important because Texas A&M Health Science Center had some medical education programs in Round Rock, and there was no desire to compete with that institution for state funds. Moreover, UT Austin had experienced significant decreases in state appropriations per student and did not want to seek state funds for a new medical school in competition with other campus needs.

Shine's financial plan was based on the important role Seton was playing not only in supporting the residency programs, but also in supporting substantial numbers of clinical faculty who taught residents and could teach medical students at the new medical school, similar to their instruction of students from the UT Medical Branch. This support was in the range of $45 million to $50 million per year. Shine concluded that the new medical school would require additional initial funding of $65 million annually (appendix 17). These funds would provide salary and other forms of support for faculty members in basic sciences, the Dean's Office, and departmental chairs. Some of these individuals might already be on the UT Austin campus in science departments and would require compensation for a portion of their time, but other new faculty would also be required. Funds would also be needed for chairs and vice chairs of clinical departments who might supervise faculty in the Seton System for academic purposes but who would also be full-time university employees. Among these individuals were the medical school Dean and other Associate Deans, as well as the necessary infrastructure for the administration of the medical school. Finally, there needed to be funding for the construction of new facilities to support the medical school.

Although philanthropy would be an important source of income for the school, it was unlikely to contribute a significant amount of funding for operations. Philanthropists customarily endow programs, research, and endowed faculty positions. However, the income from an endowed chair will, in most cases, pay for only a portion of that individual's salary.

With start-up funds from the state legislature excluded, and philanthropy, while central to the overall mission, not contributing to operations, the remaining sources for potential funding were the Board of Regents, local tax support, and industry funding or returns from patents and licensing. The latter was unlikely to be significant for a number of years. With strong support from Cigarroa, an initial proposal was considered for Board of Regents funding. Initially, this was $25 million per year, with no definite end date. Ultimately, the $25 million was translated into a percentage of AUF so that it could grow over time; UT Austin was receiving 45 percent of AUF annually. At least $25 million would be provided annually by increasing the figure to 48 percent of the AUF and could grow as the total amount of AUF increased. The other potential source of funding was property taxes assessed by Central Health. This idea had initially been considered prior to the recession in early 2008 and was now revived. Senator Watson had carried the legislation that established the hospital district and worked very closely with the Board of Managers over the years. Clarke Heidrick, in his role as Chair of the Board of Managers and as Chair of the Chamber of Commerce, saw both the opportunities and challenges of obtaining increases in tax revenue. Senator Watson suggested that he would like to see the amount of money made available by the Board of Regents closer to 50 percent of the total amount of additional needs to finance the medical school. The UT System proposal was then increased to a minimum of $25 million without limit and $5 million annually for eight years of PUF funding to be used in recruiting new faculty. This resulted in a total of $30 million and left $35 million as the requirement for the Central Health contribution.

On May 3, 2012, the Board of Regents adopted a motion creating and providing funding for the development of a medical school in Austin (appendix 20). The motion read: (1) commit to the development of a medical school in Austin; (2) commit additional AUF monies to the creation of a medical school at UT Austin equal to the greater of $25 million annually or a 3 percent increase in the annual AUF distribution to UT Austin from 45 to 48 percent; and (3) approve the allocation of $5 million in STARs recruiting monies annually for eight years to UT Austin as additional support to create the medical school at UT Austin. The resolution by Vice Chair Steve Hicks moved that the financial commitments of the Board of Regents be contingent upon the continuation of the Seton Healthcare Family's support of graduate medical education residency programs and clinical faculty positions at current or increased levels and the availability of reliable and continuing funding of $35 million annually from local community sources for the direct support of a medical school at UT Austin. He also moved that the Board review the funding streams to support the medical school ten years after its establishment, consistent with the Board's fiduciary responsibilities.

CENTRAL HEALTH TAX RATE

Like hospital districts across the State of Texas, Central Health was charged with providing healthcare for indigent Travis County residents. It had taxing authority of 7.5 cents per $100 assessed value. While Central Health could increase the tax rate by a small amount without the approval of Travis County voters, it became clear that pursuing the goals of "10 in 10" would require an additional property tax increase of 5.0 cents per $100 assessed value. This would require voter approval and would bring the Central Health tax rate to 12.9 cents per $100 assessed value. Hospital district tax rates in Dallas and Houston were in the range of 25 to 27 cents per $100 assessed value, which was considerably higher than in Travis County, even with the tax rate increase.

The timeliness of events was particularly enhanced by the State of Texas's receipt of a Medicaid 1115 Waiver in December 2011. The Waiver consisted of two parts. The largest proportion, in the first two to three years of the Waiver, was to provide funding for uncompensated care across the state. This was because the state had moved to managed care of Medicaid patients rather than the previous fee-for-service system. The change made expenditures under managed care ineligible for federal matching monies. The Waiver made up for this loss of revenue. The second portion was called the Delivery System Reform Incentive Payment. These monies became available to eligible healthcare providers to improve care of indigent patients across the full range of health services. This could include new clinics, new programs in mental health or cancer care, or combinations of new or expanded services. To obtain these funds, eligible entities like the hospital district had to make tax money available, which was matched by the federal government under the Waiver. The match was a very good one, in that every dollar of tax money spent on indigent care could be matched by $1.46 in federal funds. As a consequence, a 5.0 cent increase in the Central Health tax rate would bring in approximately $125 million to the hospital district. With federal approval of proposed programs, these monies could be effectively used to meet a number of the "10 in 10" goals, particularly those related to cancer and mental health. Annually, $35 million could be made available from Central Health for the medical school while still providing another $90 million for a wide variety of other programs.

These developments also affected the delivery model for healthcare in Travis County. As previously noted, the Community Care Collaborative (CCC) between Central Health and Seton was available to receive the federal match to Central Health's expenditures, which was approximately $125 million annually. The CCC would then disburse the funds to appropriate sources. This included monies to community clinics, which could be expanded, and to new clinics, the medical school, and the new Seton Hospital to pay for uncompensated care. None of the funds would pay for capital expenditures, such as the new Seton Teaching Hospital, or facilities for the new medical school.

THE SOUTH TEXAS CONNECTION

Although the UT System had two academic campuses in South Texas, one in Brownsville and the other in Edinburg, there was no medical school in this heavily populated area. For over thirty years, the region's community and political leadership had strongly argued for a medical school. In the late nineties, the Texas Legislature was convinced to establish a greater presence for medical education in South Texas through the creation of a regional academic health center. The state provided funding for two buildings in Harlingen and a research facility in Edinburg. All these activities were the responsibility of UTHSC–San Antonio. As early as 1998, the institution rotated as many as forty to sixty medical students annually for third- and fourth-year clerkships in South Texas. During the 2011 legislative session, UT System Regents were authorized to start a medical school in South Texas when appropriate. As previously noted, the Coordinating Board asserted in 2002 that additional medical schools in the state should be created in underserved areas, such as South Texas and West Texas. Since that time, Texas Tech created a medical school in El Paso. The Regents became increasingly concerned about the limitation of resources for programs in South Texas. Led by Chair Powell, who was born in Weslaco, Texas, and Regent Ernest Aliseda, from McAllen, the Board approved $30 million in funding for a South Texas initiative on August 25, 2009. The monies included not only support for additional programs in undergraduate education but also $10 million for a "smart hospital," which was ultimately built in Harlingen, and $3 million to support residency programs in the region.

For decades, the development of academic campuses in South Texas had been limited by their ineligibility for the use of PUF from the UT System. Multiple efforts to provide continuing funding for the campuses, UT Brownsville and UT–Pan American, had been unsuccessful. In the fall of 2010, Steve Collins, an experienced attorney in the UT System's Office of Governmental Relations, proposed that the UT System resolve this conundrum by merging the two academic campuses into a new university. He pointed out that the creation of such a new university by a two-thirds vote of the Texas Legislature could include eligibility for PUF. It was also noted that a medical school could be started at this newly created university in South Texas. Chancellor Cigarroa, supported by Chair Powell, moved expeditiously to implement Collins's plan. Ultimately, specific plans for a new medical school at the merged institution proceeded. This development was crucial to the simultaneous and successful development of the medical school in Austin. The political storm that might have been created by establishing a medical school in Austin ahead of long-standing efforts to establish a medical school in South Texas was averted. Ultimately, the two new medical schools were established essentially simultaneously, and both received preliminary accreditation in the same year. Although the political leadership in South Texas continued to assert that Regental financial support was far more generous in Austin than in South Texas, the Regents did commit an additional $10 million per year over ten years to the creation of the medical school in South Texas.

A NEW TEACHING HOSPITAL

Brackenridge Hospital was deteriorating rapidly and inadequate to serve as a modern teaching hospital. Seton and Central Health agreed that the costs of all needed renovations and repairs—including leaky roofs and out-of-date operating rooms, patient rooms, and HVAC systems and other technology—were so high that it was far better to invest in a new hospital. An expert consultation obtained by Senator Watson, from national health leaders Drs. Mitchell Rabkin and Jordan Cohen, confirmed this belief. Seton and its parent Ascension agreed to provide $250 million toward the construction of a new hospital and committed to raising an additional $50 million in philanthropy for the facility. The best location for the new hospital was near the new medical school on a site at UT Austin. The estimated cost of constructing the hospital subsequently rose to $310 million.

THE CAMPAIGN FOR CENTRAL HEALTH PROPOSITION 1

One of the important features of the 1115 Waiver was that healthcare could be paid not only for Medicaid patients but for other individuals who were medically indigent. Governance of the CCC was shared between Seton and Central Health. However, funds to the CCC would be used as part of the obligation that Central Health had to the medical school. The medical school's responsibilities included care in the hospital and in community clinics, both of which the CCC would fund. When the UT System announced, on May 3, 2012, its commitment to allocate $30 million per year for eight years, and at least $25 million annually thereafter, Senator Watson announced an effort to pass Central Health Proposition 1, which would allow the hospital district to raise its tax rate by 5.0 cents per $100 assessed value.

The Central Health election was set for November 2012. Because it was the date of a presidential election, it was expected to bring out a large number of voters to decide the fate of Proposition 1. Senator Watson organized a broad-based campaign in favor of the proposition and enlisted more than forty community groups to endorse it. He spoke and interacted with very large numbers of individuals and groups on the merits of Proposition 1. Representatives of the UT System, including Shine, Thomas, and Provost Leslie, often participated in these meetings to provide information, although they did not specifically endorse the ballot measure. Important groups such as the Chamber of Commerce, AARO,

DAA, and others endorsed the proposition. Watson's message empha-sized that the "10 in 10" program had the potential to deliver a wide range of health and economic benefits to the region, such as a greater supply of doctors in specialty care and research spin-offs. This broad-based strat-egy was attractive to many groups. In an article on October 8, 2011, the staff of the *Austin American-Statesman* reported that Republican Gov-ernor Rick Perry "supports the concept" because a medical school would help the region move closer to becoming the "next Silicon Valley."[2]

Of particular importance was the effort by Senator Watson to ob-tain the support of UT Austin President Bill Powers, who previously had significant concerns about starting and funding a new medical school. In a series of meetings with Powers, Watson made it clear that he could not move forward on the "10 in 10" program without Powers's support. In his State of the University address in September 2011, Pow-ers gave such support and indicated his commitment to the establish-ment of a "world-class" medical school (appendix 23).

CENTRAL HEALTH SUPPORT

On August 15, 2012, the Central Health Board of Managers adopted a resolution in support of a tax ratification election, as follows: "Central Health will seek voter approval for an ad valorem tax rate of $0.129 per $100 valuation for the 2013 tax year with the express intent and goal of committing increased revenues to improve healthcare in Travis County, including support for a new medical school consistent with the mission of Central Health, a site for a new teaching hospital, trauma services, specialty medicine such as cancer care, community-wide health clinics, training for physicians, nurses and other healthcare pro-fessionals, primary health, behavioral healthcare, prevention and well-ness programs, and/or to obtain federal matching funds for healthcare services" (appendix 21).

Because of all the prior work, there was little well-organized op-position to Proposition 1. The final text of the proposition read, "Approving the ad valorem tax rate of $0.129 per $100 valuation in Central Health, for the 2013 tax year, a rate that exceeds the district's rollback tax rate. The proposed ad valorem tax rate exceeds the ad valorem tax rate most recently adopted by the district by $0.05 per $100 valuation; funds will be used for improved healthcare in Travis County, including support for a new medical school consistent with the mission of Central Health, a site for a new teaching hospital, trauma services, specialty medicine such as cancer care, community-wide health clinics, training for physicians, nurses and other healthcare professionals, primary care, behavioral and mental healthcare, prevention and wellness programs, and/or to obtain federal matching funds for healthcare services."[3] The recently received Texas Medicaid Waiver allowed a significant federal match for these monies.

Subsequent concerns were raised that a Central Health tax increase to support a medical school was inconsistent with the mission and statutory authority of the hospital district. However, the preponderance of legal and policy opinions held that such funding was appropriate so long as the medical school helped advance the mission of the hospital district in providing care for the medically indigent.

Executive Vice Chancellor Shine and Vice Chancellor Thomas made several previous efforts to include St. David's HealthCare in the developments at the new medical school. In meetings with the CEO of the Austin region for HCA Healthcare, which included St. David's, he reiterated a desire to participate but limited his interest in residents and/or fellows in cardiology and other specific programs in areas where St. David's sought to substantially increase its economic and clinical advantages. At one point, the St. David's CEO offered to provide a onetime payment of $20 million as part of St. David's participation in the school. While this was a significant amount of money, it was substantially less than the $40 million to $50 million a year that Seton was spending in support of UT-sponsored residency education and faculty programs.

Three weeks prior to the Central Health vote on Proposition 1, St. David's executive David Huffstutler and his St. David's colleagues met with Chancellor Cigarroa, Shine, Thomas, and Burgdorf. At that time, St. David's leadership indicated their strong support for the medical school but urged that Central Health provide more direct financial support of St. David's programs in caring for medically indigent patients. There was no disclosure or suggestion that they would not support or, indeed, oppose Central Health Proposition 1.

A major surprise just before the November 6, 2012, election was a public announcement by Huffstutler that St. David's Healthcare opposed Proposition 1, without any prior notification to the Chancellor of this abrupt change of position. Huffstutler emphasized that St. David's supported the creation of a new medical school but did not support the increase in the tax rate. Most knowledgeable observers interpreted Huffstutler's position as largely arising from unhappiness with the lack of monies available to St. David's from federal funds flowing to the hospital district through the 1115 Medicaid Waiver. There had been active discussions between Central Health and St. David's about Central Health/CCC payment to St. David's from Waiver proceeds to support St. David's costs of providing care to the medically indigent. However, no agreement was reached with Central Health as to the required financial contribution St. David's must make to participate in the waiver program to derive the federal match.

St. David's announcement that it would not support Central Health Proposition 1 produced a number of vigorous observations on local blogs that accused "a private, for-profit healthcare system as putting their bottom line over the health of our community right here in Travis County."[4] The blogs pointed out that St. David's was controlled by the Hospital Corporation of America (HCA), a for-profit hospital system that controlled 163 hospitals across the country. The argument became very political, and the bloggers emphasized that HCA was owned by Bain Capital, a private equity firm created by Mitt Romney. Central Health, which had been accused of failing to provide adequate funding to St. David's for indigent care, argued that it had given St. David's significant opportunities to participate in the Medicaid 1115 Waiver but that St. David's had not agreed to make the required financial commitment. The St. David's financial commitment would have been matched by substantial amounts of federal money.

CAMPAIGN ISSUES

There were two principal objections to Proposition 1, the motion to increase taxes for Central Health in support of Watson's "10 in 10" initiative. The first was based on the concept that UT could afford to build a
medical school because of the size of its endowment and the profit derived from its football program. The principal protagonist of this was
Rob Moshein, of Austin, who argued that because UT had a $7 billion
endowment and the football team made a $50 million profit, it "can af-
ford the local medical school."[5] Moshein indicated that he was in favor of a UT medical school but "will vote against the proposed tax
increase pitched as vital to fulfilling such aims." The UT System responded through Controller and Associate Vice Chancellor Randy
Wallace, who explained that the payout from AUF and PUF monies invested could not exceed 7 percent of the average market value, which
was approximately $14.4 billion in the year that ended August 31, 2011.
Approximately $506 million was distributed in 2011, with the UT Sys-
tem gaining about $350 million (one-third of the $506 million went to
Texas A&M). The Austin campus would receive approximately 45 percent of the UT System's monies, nearly $158 million. The remaining
monies were required to pay debt service on certain bonds backed by
PUF monies and initiatives that benefited the UT System as a whole.
The *Austin American-Statesman*, in reviewing these assertions, indicated that $4 million had been transferred from the athletic programs
for various academic programs over a six-year period from school year
2005–2006 to 2010–2011. The *Statesman* agreed with Moshein's estimate
about the size of the endowment and the profit from UT Austin's football program, but rated his proposal half true because it could not be
"siphoned off for a medical school—year after year—without reducing
existing commitments."[6]

The other major opposition to Proposition 1 came from those
who believed that the hospital district did not have the right to raise
taxes for the purposes described. A lawsuit was filed in the U.S. District Court, Western District of Texas, that "alleges Central Health violated the Voting Rights Act by failing to submit ballot language to the

U.S. Department of Justice." Central Health responded through Christie Garbe, its Vice President for Planning and Communication, who
stated, "Central Health had a preclearance letter from the U.S. Department of Justice approving ballot language." She particularly cited, in
the Department of Justice statement, "the Attorney General does not
interpose any objection to the specification as charges" that apply to the
proposition. [7]

On October 24, 2012, Central Health responded to a St. David's letter that alleged that it had been shut out of participation in the CCC,
and that Central Health's plans to use funds intended for healthcare by
low-income and uninsured residents of Travis County would instead be
used to help fund the building of the medical school. The hospital district stated that the statement by the St. David's CEO, that there were
no opportunities to participate in the 1115 Medicaid Waiver under the
same or similar conditions in Central Texas as Seton, was not true. It
claimed that Seton and other partners "have attempted to work with St.
David's for many months to bring them into the discussion regarding
the development of the integrated delivery system model and the Medicaid Waiver. St. David's participation in this unprecedented community effort is needed. However, a true partnership is not possible without the commitment, and this includes bringing financial resources to
the table."[8] The hospital district's statements went on to indicate that
the CCC had been established to support clinics and the teaching hospital. But because there would be investing of significant public tax dollars, "the agency must maintain majority interest in the CCC in order
to protect the interest of the taxpayers." The hospital district added, "A
basic premise established at the beginning of the discussions on the
development of the CCC was that all participating partners contribute resources to its development. St. David's maintains that their indigent care services meet this requirement, thus entitling them to additional funding from this effort. Central Health and Seton have both
contributed significant resources; tax dollars from Central Health, and
$250 million [ultimately became $310 million] from Seton to build a
new teaching hospital to replace the current University Medical Center Brackenridge Hospital, as well as the significant annual GME fund-

ing Seton provides valued indigent care services and is adding to that commitment the funding of new assets for the benefit of the community." The Central Health statement goes on to point out that "under the 1115 Waiver the federal government will match $1.46 for every $1.00 raised locally which will fund projects after they meet measurable objectives to transform the healthcare delivery system. The passage of Proposition 1 will allow the community to bring the maximum amount of federal funds available back to our own community." Central Health concluded their statement by encouraging St. David's to "rejoin the discussion in order to fulfill our vision to deliver more cost-effective and comprehensive healthcare for those most in need of our care."[9]

MEDIA COVERAGE

The media closely covered this aspect of the Proposition 1 debates. In addition, at least one organization in support of Proposition 1 also pointed out that "St. David's is controlled by HCA, a gigantic corporation that controls 163 hospitals across the country and is owned by— wait for it—Bain Capital, the private equity firm started by Mitt Romney."[10] The allegation was that "a private for-profit healthcare system has put their bottom line over the health of our community right here in Travis County."[11]

Prior to the election of 2012, Steve Leslie sent a message to the faculty and staff of UT Austin. He specifically noted, "The University may not take a position on the November 6 referendum."[12] He went on to say, however, that as Provost he could outline the benefits to the university, the community, and particularly the impact of Senator Watson's "10 Goals in Ten Years" proposal. He also pointed out that the Board of Regents had expressed their commitment to the medical school by "commitment to increase UT Austin's allocation of the AUF by at least $25 million annually. An amount that could grow over time and could not decrease. Additionally, the Board of Regents have committed $5 million for each of the school's first eight years to help with recruitment and start-up." Leslie emphasized that the school would be "an innovative, interdisciplinary, inter-professional, and community-based model."[13]

During the campaign for Proposition 1 in Austin, the *Austin American-Statesman* pointed out that "it was [Senator] Watson who helped make it possible for Central Health to hold a tax election. He authored 2007 legislation that gave the agency overseeing healthcare for the needy Travis County residents broader taxing, contracting and other powers than other hospital districts in the state."[14] The *Statesman* went on to say that there were "some people who questioned Senator Watson's ties to Central Health. For one thing, Central Health has paid Senator Watson's law firm Brown, McCarroll LLP, $262,675 since May for legal work on the '10-in-10' plan and other matters."[15] The *Statesman* reported that four out-of-state ethical experts agreed that there had been no unethical behavior.

DPRI REVISITED

In October 2012, just prior to the Proposition 1 election, the role of the DPRI was again raised by the Dell Foundation. On October 10, 2012, Provost Leslie responded to their questions by emphasizing that UT Austin was "recruiting now for a DPRI director."[16] He went on to say, "It makes sense to move DPRI to the medical school, but more sense to have DPRI as a centerpiece for research that creates synergies between the academic campus and the medical school. So, we plan to salvage DPRI as an interdisciplinary unit that extends and expands reach from basic research to translational research on core topics related to pediatrics."[17] Leslie reiterated that "DPRI is and will be a crown jewel of Austin and UT Austin as a research center. We will have a very progressive timeline. Let me say also that DPRI is now a core priority of the university and will connect with the Dell Children's Hospital in a way that has it poised for aggressive expansion as we launch the medical school." Leslie noted that if the medical school was started after the election, the teaching hospital and the first two medical school buildings (a research building and a classroom/administrative building) would be built in the vicinity of Brackenridge Hospital. However, the area around DPRI and Dell Children's Hospital will be of core importance as we build out pediatric research and training associated with the medical school." He noted that some of the core priorities for DPRI currently included cancer and nutrition/obesity and their effects, which could be the foundations around which the medical school would strongly position DPRI as a center.

CHANCELLOR'S SUPPORT

On November 1, 2012, Cigarroa released a Chancellor's message in which he emphasized that "the UT System is on the verge of a once in a generation milestone—establishing a medical school at UT Austin (appendix 22). The medical school at UT Austin would be the first and only comprehensive research-intensive school of medicine on an academic campus in Texas. Such a move would complement many of UT Austin's programs, including natural science, nursing, pharmacy, and engineering. We have a unique opportunity right now to design a medical school that is a research-intensive institution, combined with strong community based educational programs."[18] The Chancellor emphasized that a school of medicine at UT Austin would enhance the university's reputation and ability to compete for the very best faculty. While emphasizing that the university could not take a position on Proposition 1, Cigarroa further outlined "great benefits to the local community of a medical school at UT Austin."[19] He reiterated the Regental financial support for the school and the actions of other communities to tax themselves in order to allow UT Austin to have a medical school.

Key to the passage of the proposition was the support of UT Austin President Powers (appendix 23). Although the Huffstutler pronouncement opposing Proposition 1 produced great anxiety among its supporters, the proposition passed by a 55 percent to 45 percent positive vote by the Travis County electorate. The breakdown was as follows: 186,128 for (54.67 percent), 154,308 against (45.33 percent).

CHAPTER 7

CREATING THE MEDICAL SCHOOL

As soon as the results of the November election were known, plans for the creation of the medical school began. Provost Leslie almost immediately appointed Robert Messing and Sue Cox to begin planning for the opening of the school. Under their leadership, a steering committee was established, and a number of working groups were organized (appendix 15). All aspects of the new medical school were considered, with special emphasis on its curriculum. Very early on, Dr. Cox led an effort to create a unique curriculum that would provide only one year of pre-clinical sciences, followed by a one-year clinical clerkship. Instead of a traditional clerkship, the third year would be devoted either to additional degrees, such as master of business administration or master of public health, or to research activity. For a limited number of students, it would be possible to omit the third-year curriculum and directly participate in the fourth-year program, with graduation after three years of medical school. A search was quickly undertaken for a Founding Dean who fit the vision for the school (appendices 25 and 26).

MEDICAL SCHOOL NAMING

The Dell Foundation offered a $50 million gift to the medical school with the understanding that the school would be named the Dell Medical School. Although the gift was not as substantial as those typically offered for the naming of major academic medical schools, it was deemed appropriate by the leadership of the UT System and the Board of Regents, based on the multiple long-standing contributions of the Dell Foundation to UT Austin and to advance health in the community. Michael and Susan Dell had previously given approximately $100 million to the university for a variety of programs, as well as $25 million for the Dell Pediatric Hospital (to which they subsequently added $13 million). In addition, it was clear they would also likely make a significant contribution to what became the Dell Seton Medical Center at the University of Texas, with the latter serving as the major teaching hospital for the medical school.

MICHAEL & SUSAN DELL FOUNDATION (DELL FOUNDATION) CHALLENGE GRANT

The Dell Foundation announced, on January 27, 2015, a challenge grant of $25 million to help Seton raise $50 million for the new 211-bed teaching hospital under construction at 15th and Red River Streets. Community leader Pete Winstead agreed to head the efforts to raise additional monies for the Dell Seton Medical Center at the University of Texas, which opened in May 2017. Construction of the hospital required a site close to the new medical school. The Board of Regents agreed to lease land for sixty years to Central Health for the construction of the new teaching hospital. Central Health subsequently leased the land on a long-term basis to Seton for the construction of a teaching hospital. The agreement allows for two additional ten-year periods after the sixty years, subject to the provisions of the lease. Seton, aided by philanthropy, constructed the new teaching hospital. However, it is subject to the terms of its sublease with Central Health providing that the purposes and functions of the hospital are consistent with the goals of Central Health. This gave Central Health some degree of control over future uses of the hospital.

MEDICAL SCHOOL BUILDINGS

Plans proceeded for the erection of three new medical school buildings, which included an academic education building (Health Learning Building), a research building (Health Discovery Building), and a clinical/physician office building (Health Transformation Building). A parking garage was also built to support the research and clinical/physician office buildings. Construction of the academic building was completed in advance of the matriculation of the first medical students in 2016, and the other two buildings were completed the following year.

AFFILIATION AGREEMENTS

Essential to the establishment of the Dell Medical School was a Memorandum of Understanding (MOU) between UT Austin, Central Health, Seton Healthcare Family, and the CCC. The CCC had been established in a separate agreement between Central Health and Seton as a not-for-profit entity to be "the main vehicle through which they will invest in new medical resources and services in Travis County for the indigent and Medical Access Program (MAP) populations and to transition into an integrated delivery system (IDS)" (appendix 24). Key provisions of the MOU provided that Seton would build and operate a new teaching hospital that would be part of Seton and Central Health's indigent and charity care safety network. It was understood that Seton and Central Health, through the CCC, would expand medical services in Travis County. UT Austin would build and operate the new medical school, with a focus on patient-centered interprofessional education and healthcare, and leading-edge basic translational research to advance the quality of healthcare. Seton was affiliated with the medical school to support faculty and train students and residents. The teaching hospital would improve and expand the medical services in Travis County available to indigent and MAP populations. Central Health and the CCC would incorporate the medical school's faculty, students, and residents into the integrated delivery system.

There were two critically important foundational Affiliation Agreements negotiated to ensure the adequate ongoing support and funding necessary to start and sustain the new medical school. The first agreement, between UT Austin, Central Health, and the CCC, was signed in August 2014 to secure the long-term annual $35 million payment from Central Health to UT Austin for permitted investments. The Central Health funding also met the requirement for ongoing local community support included in the Board of Regents motion authorizing the creation and funding of the new medical school. Permitted investments included the provision of direct operating support to UT Austin to be used in its discretion to facilitate and enhance (1) the development, accreditation, and ongoing operation of the UT Austin Dell Medical School and its administrative infrastructure; (2) the recruitment, retention, and work of the UT Austin Dell Medical School faculty, residents, medical students, researchers, administrators, staff, and other clinicians; and (3) other related activities and functions as described in the agreement.

A number of individuals in the community argued that the annual $35 million permitted investment payment should be used only to directly improve healthcare delivery to medically indigent individuals. They argued that Central Health had no right to use the monies for any other purpose. However, it was clear that when voters approved Central Health's Proposition 1, they voiced their desire to support the medical school directly and provided that UT, in its "discretion," could use the monies for a variety of purposes. Among these were medical school operations, clinical services, training of future physicians, the discovery of new knowledge, and making medical innovations available at the bedside. The proper use of the $35 million annual payment is currently in litigation.

The second foundational agreement for the new medical school was signed in October 2014. UT Austin, UT System, and Seton entered into a long-term Affiliation Agreement that outlined joint educational, clinical, and research activities of the partners in the Central Texas region. Seton agreed to continue its long-term support of UT undergraduate and graduate medical education programs. UT Austin and Seton agreed that UT Austin would not start a new material clinical program with Seton competitors in Central Texas without first offering Seton a right of first opportunity to participate.

It took many months of regular deliberations and meetings to discuss and finalize the two foundational affiliation agreements among the partners. Shine, Thomas, Cox, and Leslie were the primary negotiators on the UT side, with Greg Fenves, the Provost at UT Austin, and Patti Ohlendorf, UT General Counsel, also participating. Hartman and LaFrey were the primary Seton negotiators, while Young Brown led the Central Health team. Everyone represented the interests of their organizations well, while working diligently and collaboratively to establish sound foundations to ensure the success of the medical school and expand and improve the healthcare delivery system in the region.

THE CATHOLIC CHURCH/MEDICAL SCHOOL CONUNDRUM

The creation of the Dell Medical School with Seton as its primary clinical partner and principal teaching hospital exacerbated concerns of the mid-1990s about the impact of Catholic doctrine on patient care and, now, on medical education and research. On July 9, 2013, an organization called Americans United for Separation of Church and State sent a letter to UT Austin President Bill Powers and the members of the Central Health Board of Managers. In the letter, the organization challenged the relationship of Central Health and Seton in providing healthcare services to Travis County. It argued that a Catholic healthcare organization that was restricted from providing certain medical services by the Ethical and Religious Directives for Catholic healthcare services was engaged with a governmental public hospital district charged with "providing healthcare services to Travis County." The issues revolved primarily around reproduction issues, including abortion, contraception, and sterilization.[1]

The hospital district responded that it had arranged for pregnant women desiring sterilization at the time of delivery, and that other women seeking contraception and/or sterilization, though they were not pregnant, were to be cared for at a St. David's facility. A full range of reproductive medical services would be available at St. David's ambulatory care sites. Abortions, when medically indicated, contraception, and tubal ligation would be available at St. David's Hospital and other facilities operated by the medical school. Residents in the OB/GYN program at Seton currently also rotate through St. David's facilities, where they have these experiences.

The UT System indicated that the medical school would also be responsible for the instruction of students' full range of issues for end-of-life care. While at Seton facilities, they would be exposed to effective teaching in this area. They would also have rotations at other institutions, both inpatient and outpatient, where different philosophies toward reproductive issues and end-of-life care existed. It is not unusual for students and residents to have multiple exposures to different philosophies related to these complex issues.

The medical school did not anticipate any difficulty with accreditation issues arising out of potential church/state conflicts. The school had confidence that the medical school curriculum was entirely their responsibility and would be consistent with LCME requirements. Initial accreditation was accomplished and expeditiously approved for matriculation of the first medical school class in July 2016.

UT leadership expressed a strong belief that public monies would be used appropriately for the care of patients and the education of students. On November 19, 2012, Shine stated, "Many medical schools with affiliations with Catholic hospitals are accredited so long as the full range of appropriate educational opportunities are available to students. Stem cell research can be conducted at a UT Austin medical school in collaboration with a wide variety of institutions locally and nationally. The hospital district has paid for services from a variety of sources including the OB/GYN services at St. David's to provide a full range of services. Students do not directly comply with directives. The care of patients is determined by the attending physicians who presumably are influenced by institutional policies. The students concerned about learning in this environment may learn at another healthcare facility, including St. David's. Please note that St. David's has participated in student and resident education and has said that it supports the medical school, just not the funding mechanism."[2] Though no subsequent legal actions have been taken since the July 2013 letter from Americans United for Separation of Church and State, many anticipate that these issues will resurface in the future.

SEARCH COMMITTEE FOR DEAN OF THE MEDICAL SCHOOL

A search committee was established to recruit the Dean of the medical school. The search committee consisted of eighteen educators, community leaders, health professionals, and students, and was chaired by Robert Messing, who had become Vice Provost for Biomedical Sciences and the Henry M. Burlage Centennial Professor of Pharmacy.

Dr. Clay Johnston, a distinguished faculty member at the University of California, San Francisco, was selected as the first Dean (appendices 26 and 27). He had a very successful career studying the epidemiology and management of stroke at UCSF. His enthusiasm for the new school was based on his interest in promoting value-based healthcare with strong community interactions, with an emphasis on new care delivery methodologies. He emphasized these concepts in articulating the mission of the institution to potential students. The first students matriculated in July 2016.

Shine was succeeded by Dr. Raymond Greenberg as Executive Vice Chancellor for Health Affairs in September 2013. However, Shine remained for an additional two years as a Special Adviser to the Chancellor, with the responsibility of assisting with the development of the Dell Medical School, as well as the medical school in South Texas. Shine formally retired from the UT System in July 2015. Thomas remained as Vice Chancellor and Counsel for Health Affairs, with a specific responsibility for overseeing the two medical schools and coordinating the relationships between the schools and their academic campuses. This was a particularly challenging responsibility, given that the UT System had not previously experienced a medical school as part of an academic campus.

CONCLUSION

The establishment of the Dell Medical School on the UT Austin campus was a major landmark after more than 135 years of separation between the academic campus and its medical branch. The separation of the two entities was established through a political process in 1881 and withstood a number of attempts to bring the Galveston campus to Austin over the subsequent century. Curiously enough, the separation of medical schools from academic campuses continued as the standard configuration for all other University of Texas medical schools, as well as other medical schools in the state, until the Board of Regents simultaneously established the UT Austin and UTRGV medical schools.

Although the leadership of the UT System strongly supported the establishment of an Austin medical school, it was the determination of Senator Watson and the local community that ultimately made it happen. Seton supported the training of medical residents for over eighty years and the education of medical students, principally from the UT Medical Branch, for thirty years. Seton had also hired a significant number of faculty to teach residency and medical students in the clinical disciplines, creating an opportunity for a medical school. The Brackenridge Hospital, which eventually became the Dell Seton Medical Center at the University of Texas, offered an essential teaching hospital for the new medical school.

It was ultimately the fortitude and courage of many leaders, the community, the visionary leadership of Senator Watson, and the unprecedented approval of a property tax by the voters of Travis County that led to the successful creation of the medical school. The Board of Regents, Seton, and Central Health provided the key ongoing funding needed to create and sustain the school.

Establishing the UT Austin Dell Medical School was a major accomplishment, particularly in view of the lack of initial enthusiasm and, at times, opposition from some academic leaders at UT Austin. However, the success of the academic campus, with its substantial biomedical research and health professional education programs, made the creation of a new medical school on the campus logical and extremely beneficial. Key roles were played by UT System Regent and Chair of the Board James Huffines; Greg Hartman and Charles Barnett of the Seton Healthcare Family; Clarke Heidrick and Rosie Mendoza of the Central Health Board; Patricia Young Brown, CEO of Central Health; Pete Winstead, Austin community activist; UT System Chancellors Mark Yudof and Cigarroa; Shine and Thomas; and Janet Mountain of the Dell Foundation.

The new medical school is positioned for unprecedented achievements as part of a great university. Outstanding leadership has been provided initially by UT Austin Provost and later President Greg Fenves, former Provost and Dean of the College of Pharmacy Steve Leslie, Founding Dean Clay Johnston, and Founding Executive Vice Dean Sue Cox. The school has adopted a unique approach to the support of value-based medical care, fundamental change in the healthcare delivery model, and the recruitment of students who are committed to its mission.

As the first medical school created on an AAU campus in decades, the Dell Medical School offers extraordinary promise for the future. Its establishment, based on the taxation of Travis County property owners to fund the long-term operation of a medical school, is unique in America. The Dell Medical School and the vast complementary expertise on the UT Austin campus will produce transformative discoveries and advancements that will improve the lives of Texans, while enhancing the economic vitality of the state.

Austin Residency Programs, Current Status of Graduate Medical Education in Austin, May 2013

Faculty and Resident numbers by program

Program	Paid Directly to Faculty	Volunteer Faculty	Residents May 2013	Residents July 2013
Child Neurology	*peds		NP	1
Craniofacial Surgery	0	6	1	1
Dermatology	5	5	6	9
Emergency Medicine	1	*surg	8	15
Family Medicine	10	1	21	21
Internal Medicine	31	28	48	48
Neurology	11	2	9	9
Obstetrics/Gynecology	20	24	19	21
Pediatrics	18	89	51	54
Pediatric Emergency Medicine	2			4
Physical Medicine & Rehabilitation	2	0	2	4
Psychiatry	26	5	24	24
Child Psychiatry	*psych		7	8
Psychosomatic Medicine	*psych		0	2
Surgery	10	23	12	15
Transitional Year	1		6	6
TOTAL	**144**	**188**	**214**	**243**

Resident Applicant Pool for 2013

	# Applicants	Plan to Interview
Dermatology	410	30
Emergency Medicine	1115	100
Family Medicine	760	100
Internal Medicine	2720	203
Neurology	227	38
Obstetrics/Gynecology	413	90
Pediatrics	951	214
Pediatric Emergency Medicine	27	
Physical Medicine & Rehabilitation	269	70
General Psychiatry	719	57
Child Psychiatry	N/A	
Psychosomatic Medicine	N/A	
Surgery	678	67
Transitional Year	684	80

Quality of 2013 Match applicants: USMLE scores Step 1 and Step 2

	USMLE Step 1 (National Mean)	USMLE Step 2 (National Mean)
Dermatology	237 (242)	**257 (252)**
Emergency Medicine	**225 (224)**	226 (237)
Family Medicine	**213 (208)**	**232 (219)**
Internal Medicine	**221 (221)**	**231 (230)**
Neurology	**222 (222)**	226 (230)
Obstetrics/Gynecology	208 (218)	**240 (233)**
Pediatrics	**225 (216)**	**241 (229)**
Phys Medicine & Rehab	Not Avail	Not Avail
General Psychiatry	209 (219)	**222 (218)**
Child Psychiatry	Not Avail	Not Avail
Surgery	**231 (227)**	**245 (239)**
Transitional Year	**250 (240)**	**238 (248)**

Bolded = above the National Mean
USMLE = United States Medical Licensing Examination
ACGME = Accreditation Council for Graduate Medical Education

UTMB 3RD AND 4TH YEAR MEDICAL STUDENTS IN AUSTIN
Third year enrollment (clerkships):
43 Austin-based third year students
61 Galveston-based students enrolled in one or more clerkships in Austin

Third Year Clerkship Capacities:
FM—2 (12 terms)
Pedi—12 (6 terms)
Surg—8 (6 terms)
Psych—15 (8 terms)
Ob/Gyn—6 (8 terms}
IM—15 (4 terms)

Fourth year enrollment (clerkships/electives):
42 Austin-based students enrolled in one or more courses in Austin
39 Galveston-based students enrolled in one or more courses in Austin
90 visiting (non-UTMB) students enrolled in one or more courses in Austin

Fourth Year Capacities:
Sr. Surgery Clerkship—4 (13 periods)
Sr. Neurology Clerkship—4 (13 periods)
Emergency Medicine Selective—4 (13 periods)
+ 38 electives

TEXAS A&M 3RD AND 4TH YEAR MEDICAL STUDENTS IN AUSTIN
Pediatrics: ~60/year (2–3 students every two weeks)
Psychiatry: 18 per year

Summit 2000, Summary of the Proceedings, November 30, 2000

Summit 2000: Better Medication Outcomes Through Healthcare Collaboration

Summary of the Proceedings
November 29-30, 2000
Barton Creek Conference Center, Austin, Texas

In November 1999, the Institute of Medicine (IOM) of the National Academy of Sciences released its report, "To Err is Human: Building a Safer Health System," on the quality of health care in the United States. The intense coverage of the report by the media suggested that the health care system in the US was failing to protect patients in its care. Patient safety was a major concern of healthcare providers and organizations in Texas before the IOM report as evidenced by a number of significant advances in this area.

Bar coded patient wristbands reduced medication errors and improved the accuracy of patients' charts at the Veterans Administration health care system and St. Luke's Episcopal Hospital in Houston; Memorial Hermann Hospital in Houston reduced the number of infants suffering blood stream- and ventilator-associated pneumonia in its NICU and the number of adverse drug events over a three-year period by fifty percent; and Scott and White Memorial Hospital in Temple implemented a plan for formalized multifunctional teams to systematically measure and improve quality and patient safety.

However, the IOM report led members of the Texas Pharmacy Congress (TPC) to the conclusion that there was clearly a need for a positive, persistent, and collaborative process to work through the issues of lack of integration, communication, and cooperation in healthcare systems, which are among the causes of problems in patient safety. The TPC is the coalition of all Texas pharmacy organizations including the state's four colleges of pharmacy, Texas Pharmacy Association, Texas Society of Health-System Pharmacists, Texas Federation of Drug Stores, and the Texas State Board of Pharmacy.

There was clearly a need for a positive, persistent, and collaborative process to work through the issues of lack of integration, communication, and cooperation in healthcare systems which are among the causes of problems in patient safety.

Consequently the TPC quickly organized a multidisciplinary steering committee to plan a summit on medication safety that would begin this collaborative process. The steering committee was comprised of TPC members and representatives of non-pharmacy organizations, including the Texas Medical Association, Texas Academy of Family Physicians, and Texas Nurses Association. According to Steven W. Leslie, Dean of the College of Pharmacy, The University of Texas at Austin, "Texas was not the first state to address the issue of patient safety, but with this Summit, Texas has the opportunity to take a leadership role."

Summit 2000 Convened To Improve Medication Safety

On November 29 and 30, 2000, 97 individuals from a broad cross section of institutional and community practice areas, including medicine, nursing, hospital administration, and pharmacy, as well as healthcare industry and consumer representatives of state health licensing boards attended *Summit 2000: Better Medication Outcomes Through Healthcare Collaboration* at Barton Creek Conference Center in Austin, Texas.

The goal of Summit 2000 was to begin to create a system that minimizes medication errors by

- Identifying ways in which statewide organizations can assist grass roots practitioners to eliminate errors in their practices,
- Promoting non-punitive error reporting among all branches of healthcare,
- Initiating open dialogue on ways to reduce errors, and
- Developing specific recommendations that can be implemented to reduce the possibility of medication errors as part of the healthcare system.

The objective of Summit 2000 was to identify the ways in which individuals and organizations could actively collaborate to reduce errors.

The objective of Summit 2000 was to identify the ways in which individuals and organizations could actively collaborate to reduce errors through education, legislation, changes in practice, and enhanced communication in an inter-professional workshop format. AstraZeneca provided support for program development and materials and

Janssen Pharmaceutica, Merck & Co, and SmithKline Beecham provided additional support.

Solutions for Improving Medication Safety

During the course of the two-day Summit, four prominent speakers offered their unique perspectives on solutions for improving medication safety, which were intended to help participants begin a comprehensive discussion of issues to formulate recommendations.

"Building A Learning Organization"

The first speaker, Josie R. Williams, M.D., MMM, CPE, Medical Director, Texas Health Quality Alliance, discussed the importance of healthcare systems becoming learning organizations. She began by providing various definitions of learning organizations from Peter Senge, author of *The Fifth Discipline*. These included "a group of people continually enhancing their capacity to create what they want to create," "one that discovers how to tap people's commitment and capacity to learn at all levels of the organization," and "one that is committed to the continuous testing of experience and transformation of that experience into knowledge."

Dr. Williams pointed out that most healthcare systems are not learning organizations and that they are not even integrated systems. While they have excellent components, such as physicians, hospitals, and technology, they are fragmented, overspecialized, have the wrong incentives, and lack understanding across specialty areas.

Most healthcare systems are not learning organizations.... They are not even integrated systems.

She described the five building blocks needed for integrated healthcare systems: an overreaching vision, which is communicated to everyone; a psychology of abundance, which means it is everyone's job to win; capability for vulnerability, (i.e. people are not afraid to admit mistakes); mutual learning from each other; and depth of leadership, which means that every individual has the leadership tools to carry out his or her projects.

To become a good learning system, Dr. Williams explained that it is necessary to examine and transform core organizational values in the areas of managing change, communication, conflict resolution, systems, vision, leadership, culture, and fundamental knowledge.

Dr. Williams concluded by stating that in a learning organization every healthcare professional is responsible for improving quality. This means that everyone has two jobs. Ninety percent of their time is spent doing their regular jobs and the remaining ten percent in improving the quality of their regular jobs. Management has the responsibility to give all professionals the tools (i.e. training and infrastructure), time, and vision to improve quality.

In a learning organization every healthcare professional is responsible for improving quality.

"Error, Stress and Teamwork in Medicine and Aviation"

David Musson, MD, MRC Fellow, The University of Texas Human Factors Research Project, The University of Texas at Austin, discussed ways to apply safety initiatives from the aviation industry to the practice of medicine. Dr. Musson described the commonality between the aviation and healthcare industries. In both, safety is a super-ordinate goal, teamwork is essential, risk varies from low to high, and threats and errors come from multiple sources. Human errors in aviation and medicine stem from human limitations, such as limited memory and processing capacities, limits imposed by stressors, fatigue, and other psychological factors, poor group dynamics, and cultural influences.

According to Dr. Musson, the aviation approach to errors has concentrated on a system approach to errors; organized development of countermeasures, such as Crew Resource Management (i.e. formalized training for aircrew in teamwork and decision making) and proceduralization (e.g., refined checklists); and research and data collection in an ongoing basis in support of safety.

One of the most significant research contributions to aviation safety was the demonstration that failures and limitations inherent in the organization's operating system predispose the best-qualified and motivated individuals and teams to err.

Aviation can provide medicine with a template for managing threats to safety and actual errors, Dr. Musson explained. This template includes:
- Understanding the history and issues in the organization,
- Diagnosing the error-inducing conditions by obtaining accurate data on current practices (including confidential reporting systems, surveys of personnel, and observations of normal practices),
- Changing the organizational culture to a safety culture that recognizes the inevitability of error and actively seeks and reduces latent threats,
- Training in effective teamwork, decision-making and error management, as well as technical aspects of the job,

3

- Providing feedback and reinforcement for effective teamwork and error management, and
- Recognizing the continuing need for accurate data on threat and error management and recurrent training in the human factors of teamwork.

Failures and limitations inherent in the organization's operating system predispose the best-qualified and motivated individuals and teams to err.

"Consumers and Medication Errors, The Delicate Balance "

Susan Jacobson, Executive Director, El Paso Child Guidance Center and a past consumer member and President of the Texas State Board of Pharmacy, focused on some of the factors contributing to medication errors that consumers can potentially affect. Her primary message was that consumers and healthcare providers have to meet each other at least half way in addressing problems of medication safety.

Ms. Jacobson offered simple steps that both patients and healthcare providers can take during professional interactions. Patients should make sure they review prescriptions and know what medications are being prescribed for themselves or their children and how to use them. They should be reminded to share with their physicians what other pharmaceuticals they may be taking. Physicians must provide prescriptions that are legible. Healthcare organizations need to institute procedures that eliminate the potential for misunderstanding prescriptions. For example, Denver County Hospital instituted a hospital-wide computer system whose primary purpose is to have all doctors electronically input their

prescriptions instead of manually writing them.

At pharmacies, consumers need to tell pharmacists what medications they are taking and what allergies they have. They need to take the time to listen to pharmacists explain how their prescription medications work and what they might experience when taking them.

However, pharmacists are suffering from "clerical work" overload and from challenging working conditions, which can interfere with patient counseling. This situation will not be changed until pharmacists and pharmacy organizations stand up and declare that they will no longer compromise the quality of their work and their licenses by accepting these conditions, Ms. Jacobson emphasized.

Consumers and healthcare providers have to meet each other at least half way in addressing problems of medication safety.

Ms. Jacobson concluded by stating that consumers need to be empowered and better informed about how to help prevent and report medication errors. On the flip side, healthcare entities responsible for patient safety need to be responsive and respectful of the consumer, which would undoubtedly raise consumer confidence.

"Medication Errors: Where Do We Go From Here?"

Joanne F. Turnbull, Ph.D, Executive Director, National Patient Safety Foundation (NPSF), which was created three years ago to raise awareness of the problem of patient safety and act as a catalyst for improving safety through education and networking addressed the

4

issue from a national perspective. Dr. Turnbull stated that the first steps in preventing medication errors are acknowledging that errors come from systems failure and identifying areas of vulnerability in healthcare systems. Preventing errors means designing safer systems of care.

Fixing the medication use system is easy, Dr. Turnbull continued. What really needs to happen is a complete cultural change on all levels of the healthcare system. This change must start on the frontlines, or "sharp-end," which includes patients and families, physicians, nurses, and pharmacists. It must continue up through all the other levels, including administration; research and education; payors; trade associations, alliances, and academic programs; government, regulators, and legal systems; pharmaceutical companies, device makers, and technology companies, who don't think they are involved in the problem; and finally the economy, media, and science. The cultures of organizations at all these levels need to be aligned to make patient safety a reality.

Fixing the medication use system is easy. What really needs to happen is a complete cultural change on all levels of the healthcare system.

Dr. Turnbull offered examples of specific cultural changes that can be made on each level. Patients and families need to be empowered to talk to providers about medication safety. The NPSF is developing a communications tool for patients on how to find a pharmacist concerned about safety. There needs to be funding for a national network of support services for victims and families of medical errors.

One of the biggest cultural barriers to improving safety is the "authority gradient" that exists on the frontline between superiors and subordinates. To overcome fear of authority, the NPSF has created cards for nurses that encourages them to "speak up" to superiors when they know an error has been made. Safety science, which deals with all the factors involved in organizational accidents or incidents (i.e., human factors, organizational factors, and technical factors), should also be integrated into every educational curriculum.

Preventing errors means designing safer systems of care.

On the administrative level, managers need new roles as communicators, translators, facilitators, and mentors and the skills to fulfill them. These will enable them to make sure top management knows what is happening on the frontline from the professionals who see problems firsthand and that those professionals, in turn, understand the organizational vision and maintain the ability to think critically and implement that vision.

Dr. Turnbull stated that there needs to be a new language for errors:
- Slips, which are errors that occur during actions guided by familiar routines and are caused by factors such as habit, interruptions, anger, anxiety, or boredom.
- Mistakes, which are errors of judgment made in unfamiliar situations with inadequate information.
- Near misses, which are errors caught before commission.

Finally, Dr. Turnbull stated that healthcare systems need to change to a culture where people like to report errors, they are rewarded for reporting them instead of penalized, and they analyze and learn

5

from errors. Recording near misses is especially important to understanding and improving the processes involved in making common errors.

Healthcare systems need to change to a culture where people like to report errors, they are rewarded for reporting them instead of penalized, and they analyze and learn from errors.

Recommendations for Action from Summit 2000 Workgroups

All Summit 2000 attendees participated in two-day workgroups that discussed "Medication Error Reduction Systems," "The Public and Medication Errors," "Performance Standards," and "Environmental Issues." Each workgroup was charged with developing recommendations for improving safety through concrete action paths. All attendees then gathered to review and prioritize the issues.

The following represents the Summit consensus on the most important issues and recommendations.

Issue: **There are disincentives for reporting errors in our culture due to fear of liability and punitive action. This leads to perpetuation of errors, systems failures, and underreporting.**

- Medication error reporting systems need to address failures and identify weaknesses in systems to reduce errors.
- Healthcare leaders should work to create a non-punitive, anonymous medication error reporting system that encourages openness, sharing of information, and a cultural shift from a 'cycle of fear' to a systems-based approach, identifying causes of errors.

- Punitive measures should remain strictly enforced for practitioners who increase errors by knowingly and intentionally overriding error-reduction systems and procedures and incentives should be developed for error reduction. Performance standards should be designed to focus on the system, not just the individual.
- Healthcare systems should provide psychological and social support counseling of practitioners to encourage reporting and error recovery.

Issue: **Systems need to track errors and monitor reporting to determine if errors are reduced.**

- A uniform baseline of measurement and a method to track trends should be included in any reporting system. Such a system must be able to address the issues of patient confidentiality and concerns about personal privacy.
- Uniform error reporting methods and definitions should be developed and promoted.
- Methods to evaluate outcomes and the effectiveness of interventions must be built into any reporting system. Access to de-identified information that can assist in error reduction must be allowed across professional practice boundaries.

Issue: **There is inadequate use of technology that could facilitate recognition of systems errors and potentials for error.**

- Healthcare leaders should develop and promote compatible technology sources to allow sharing of patient data and information, such as a shared database for drug usage with confidentiality safeguards.
- Healthcare leaders should promote new technology that would provide

6

greater information resources and less reliance on individual interpretation for practitioners, such as a smart card system containing comprehensive patient data.

- Healthcare leaders should develop interdisciplinary strategies for using technology and other initiatives to address workplace shortages across all health care disciplines.
- Healthcare leaders should redesign systems utilizing available technology in transferring the medication order from the prescriber to the patient, including:
    - electronic prescribing
    - computerized physician orders
    - scanning technology
    - pharmaceutical technology (standardized packaging)
    - integrated computer systems
    - integration of hospital and community care
    - common third-party claim forms

Issue: **Communications among and between all healthcare providers must be improved.**

- Healthcare leaders should work to improve communication among all healthcare providers. Use of current technology is one effective means to enhance communications.
- Healthcare leaders should promote quality assurance training programs, increased training, licensing and/or certification of non-licensed personnel and incorporation of training in risk management for practitioners.
- Healthcare leaders should promote training in communications techniques and team collaboration skills for students, practitioners, and patients. "Full circle" communications systems, from diagnosis to dispensing to the patient, should be incorporated to assure positive patient outcomes.
- Undergraduate and post-graduate education should incorporate

information and training on current laws and regulations for error reporting as well as systems and methods to reduce errors in practice.

- Healthcare leaders should focus on events relating to patients' transitions from community to institutional to community health care services, particularly regarding continuity of care and transfer of information.

Issue: **Public awareness and education of the patient's responsibility in health care and error reduction should be promoted.**

- Healthcare leaders should make it a priority for providers to maximize communication with their patients to improve compliance and outcomes including:
    - Standardization of information
    - Researching the most effective techniques for various demographic groups
    - Repetition of message
- Healthcare leaders should develop and implement a public relations/consumer awareness education campaign, engage consumer advocacy groups and consumers in a dialogue regarding medication errors and their role in the reduction or errors.
- Healthcare leaders should promote the investigation of the impact of the system of litigation and its effect on error reporting and reduction.
- Healthcare leaders and practitioners should communicate regularly with the media to keep them informed about the complexity of the issue.
- Reimbursement systems should take into account expenses for medication error reduction systems and other types of error reduction activities.

7

Issue: **There is a lack of coordination and collaboration between various healthcare disciplines.**

- Healthcare leaders should formalize a multidisciplinary alliance of professional organizations, regulatory agencies, and higher education institutions to have open discussions to recommend action steps to reduce medication errors. Such efforts should recognize that 'all healthcare is local' and understand that some solutions may work in one setting but not another.
- Professional associations should take the lead in promoting development of model policy manuals and standard operating procedures to address medication errors and other cross-discipline issues.
- A system for sharing best practices among disciplines must be developed and promoted.
- Healthcare leaders should work to improve management of workflow and workspace, decrease noise levels and distractions, provide private space in pharmacies for patient counseling, and delegate specific duties to pharmacy personnel.
- All practitioner groups must recognize the need to invest more resources in identification and reduction of errors, quality assurance programs and evaluation of outcomes.

The Summit concluded with reactions of a panel of representatives from different segments of the Texas healthcare community to the meeting. All panel members not only expressed unqualified agreement with the group's recommendations but enthusiasm for pursuing further dialogue and collaboration in achieving the goal of reducing medication errors.

Members of the Texas Pharmacy Congress (TPC) are continuing discussions with the various stakeholders about implementing the recommendations of the conference. Initial meetings to establish the Texas Healthcare Provider Coalition for Patient Safety for the purpose of carrying on the goals of the Summit have been held.

Note: This document is a product of the Texas Pharmacy Congress' medication error summit and does not necessarily reflect the policy or position of any person or association. Until final acceptance by each appropriate entity, this document should not be construed to establish a statement or position on the issues discussed herein by any person or entity.

Board of Regents Minutes on Expanded Role, November 12, 2003

6. **Expanded role with U. T. Austin and other organizations in medical education and health research in Austin**

PURPOSE

Dr. Guckian will lead a discussion of proposed collaborative plans for possible expanded medical education and research in Austin. No action is requested of the Board of Regents at this time. Any program or agreement requiring Regental action (for example, joint degree programs and contracts) will be presented for action at a later date.

BACKGROUND INFORMATION

The University of Texas Medical Branch at Galveston has a long history of medical service and partnership in Austin. U. T. Medical Branch–Galveston has been training residents at Brackenridge Hospital since the 1950s. The 77th and 78th Legislatures authorized U. T. Medical Branch–Galveston to spend appropriated and institutional funds to support and develop student and resident training services in Austin (General Appropriations Act, Article III, Section 7). In 2002, 106 U. T. Medical Branch–Galveston medical students performed clerkships in Austin; U. T. Medical Branch–Galveston currently has 112 medical students in clerkships in Austin. Most recently, U. T. Medical Branch–Galveston presented to the accrediting body for medical residencies, the Residency Review Committee (RRC), its plan for an Austin-based U. T. Medical Branch–Galveston Obstetrics/Gynecology residency.

U. T. Medical Branch–Galveston has entered into discussions with a number of organizations in Central Texas, with the U. T. Austin Graduate School establishing a M.D./Ph.D. program, with Seton/Brackenridge Hospital regarding expanding the number of residency programs and medical students in Austin, and with the Central Texas Veterans Healthcare System (VA System) regarding additional services provided to veterans and participating in clinical research. The U. T. Health Science Center–Houston School of Public Health likewise has entered into discussions with U. T. Austin and the Texas Department of Health regarding collaborative planning in research and education. These collaborations would complement and benefit all three U. T. com-ponent institutions. Examples include bioengineering, informatics, and expanded and diverse clinical experiences for students and residents. Eventually, these organizations, along with several others, decided to work and plan more formally. As a consequence, they formed a nonprofit association, Central Texas Institute for Research and Education in Medicine and Biotechnology (CTI). CTI is committed to the advancement and application of biomedical research and health science education in Central Texas. Members of CTI include:

- The University of Texas at Austin
- The University of Texas Medical Branch at Galveston
- The University of Texas School of Public Health at Houston
- Daughters of Charity Health Services (Seton Medical Center/Brackenridge Hospital)–Austin
- St. David's Healthcare Partnership–Austin
- Central Texas Veterans Healthcare System–Temple
- Greater Austin Chamber of Commerce

The University of Texas Health Science Center at San Antonio recently appointed an advisory representative to CTI.

EDUCATIONAL GOALS OF CTI
EXPAND HEALTH PROFESSIONAL EDUCATION IN AUSTIN
To support, enhance, and bring recognition to undergraduate and graduate medical education by

- providing a system for education of medical students and residents through affiliated in-patient facilities and clinics in Austin;
- studying community needs and providing additional residency programs to address those needs; and
- expanding access to health services to, and public health infrastructure for, citizens in Central Texas.

ESTABLISH JOINT DEGREE PROGRAMS
A jointly developed curriculum for M.D./Ph.D. (U. T. Austin and U. T. Medical Branch–Galveston) and M.D./Master of Public Health programs (U. T. Austin and U. T. Medical Branch–Galveston; U. T. Austin and U. T. School of Public Health–Houston) will be planned.

EXPAND SCHOOL OF PUBLIC HEALTH PROGRAMS
Strengthen public health activities in Austin by building relationships with other public health entities for the purpose of collaborating on meaningful and functional public health projects.

HEALTH-CARE WORKFORCE DEVELOPMENT
To collaborate, develop, and participate in the coordination of health science education and training at the community college, undergraduate, and graduate levels for the purpose of creating a supply of medical personnel to staff area medical facilities.

RESEARCH GOALS OF CTI
INCREASE MULTI-INSTITUTIONAL COLLABORATION
- Develop facilities, infrastructure, and personnel
- Joint work on clinical studies
- Develop wet lab space
- Acquire medical instrumentation
- Imaging Center (The VA System, U. T. Austin and U. T. Medical Branch–Galveston plan to install and operate an imaging center by the end of 2004.)
- Move basic science research to commercialization
- Collaborative grant writing

ENHANCE THE DEVELOPMENT OF INTELLECTUAL
PROPERTY FOR COMMERCIALIZATION
Interface with business community for the commercialization of biomedical and biotech research. Outcome of interfacing is to gain venture capital, business plans, and marketing expertise and to produce patents, products, and services.

INCREASE INFLUENCE ON PUBLIC POLICY
THROUGH EVIDENCE-BASED RESEARCH
Develop the capacity to enable researchers and public health students to collaborate and consolidate research expertise for all areas of public health. Expected outcomes are reports on the health of Texas and to translate research findings into public health policy.

APPENDIX 4

Austin Academic Health Center Proposal, August 10, 2004

AUSTIN ACADEMIC HEALTH CENTER

Considerable community interest has been expressed in the further development and expansion of medical research and education programs in Austin. Opportunities are particularly attractive in synergy with the strong research programs of The University of Texas at Austin (UT Austin) academic campus. These could take advantage of that campus's excellence in a number of areas, including engineering, computer science, pharmacy, computational science, the institute for cellular and molecular biology, the institute for neuroscience and the developing imaging center. High-quality research and educational programs conducted between an academic health center and UT Austin would enhance faculty recruiting by both institutions. Such programs would also have significant positive economic impact and expand exemplary patient care programs.

Austin has excellent hospitals and a highly-trained community of physicians who contribute to the education of medical students and post-graduate medical residents. Undergraduate medical students* at the University of Texas Medical Branch at Galveston (UTMB) already participate in teaching rotations in Austin teaching hospitals and clinics during their third and fourth years of medical school. Collaborations between UTMB and UT Austin can further enhance the education of medical students and of physician scientists. The two institutions are currently developing a combined MD/PhD program.

UTMB has a long history of involvement with academic affiliations in Austin. UTMB has also a history of facilitating the development of other UT health campuses (UT San Antonio, UT Houston). Recently, it opened a women's health hospital as part of the Brackenridge facilities in Austin and has received approval for a residency program in obstetrics and gynecology. UTMB has played an active role in the Central Texas Institute for Research & Education in Medicine & Biotechnology, an Austin based consortium devoted to the development of academic health and research programs locally. The creation of an academic health center in Austin would be managed by UTMB, in collaboration with UT Austin in a manner that could expeditiously create additional research and educational programs. A state of the art fast MRI imaging program is now under joint development by UTMB, UT Austin and the Central Texas Veterans Administration.

Substantial interest has been expressed in the creation of a four-year medical school in Austin. Such development faces very substantial challenges. The construction of facilities to educate students in basic sciences is very expensive. Resources and high-quality research programs to attract high-quality faculty to teach these students will also be costly. Considerable opposition may arise from other communities in Texas, who wish to have a medical school. The most recently established medical school, Texas Tech in El Paso has built some facilities, but not yet received operating funds. Substantial contributions from private donors or foundations would likely be required to make a medical school feasible in Austin, particularly under current state budgetary limitations.

An academic health center can be developed in Austin through a series of incremental steps which would build research, education and patient care capacity over ten to twelve years. Such an academic health center can be developed in accordance with the following principles:

A. Each component of the enterprise must be of the highest quality so as to recruit a world-class faculty and develop outstanding educational and clinical programs that are nationally recognized.

B. The academic health center should be physically located proximate to the UT Austin campus, in order to truly synergize on the capacities of each enterprise. The Mueller Airport site would be one such location, and would be ideally suited for this purpose. There are other nearby locations that could be considered. In addition, it would be convenient to primary teaching hospitals and clinics.

C. The incremental approach would include the creation and staffing of two or more research institutes, gradually expanding educational programs for undergraduate students seeking MD or MD/PhD programs and the addition of post-graduate residency training programs in the various medical specialties. These parallel developments in research and education would be intimately related to further improvements in the quality and spectrum of clinical care provided.

D. A major step in development of an academic medical center would be the establishment of a medical research institute which capitalizes on the synergy with UT Austin. Such an institute might focus on neurosciences, cancer genetics, systems biology, or other aspects of molecular medicine. Substantial support from private donors would be required to create such an institute in a relatively short period of time. The director of the institute would report to the president of UTMB for operations and to the presidents of UTMB and UT Austin with regard to program development. Faculty could be appointed to UTMB with joint appointments with UT Austin. Substantial resources would be required to attract the very best scientists and teachers to this focused enterprise to provide a high-quality research anchor for the academic health center. Gifted clinicians would be recruited as part of the translational and educational component of this focused effort, for example neurologists and geneticists. The research institute would include meeting rooms and an auditorium as part of its research and educational mission. After successful establishment of the first research institute, the second could be established in another medical field, for example the first might focus on neuroscience while the second could focus on cardiovascular research. Subsequently, additional institutes would be added to broaden the research and educational capacity. Depending on the resources available, each component could be developed in adjacent buildings on the same site.

E.   The Seton System will build and open the new Austin Children's Hospital and a related medical office building at the Mueller site by 2007. The Central Texas Veterans Administration has expressed an interest in building an inpatient/ambulatory facility on this site. Additional office space for outstanding clinical faculty could be located as part of this development. These facilities would provide a geographical base for medical students during their third and fourth year of an educational experience which would take place primarily in hospitals and in these clinic facilities. UTMB can gradually increase the number of students participating in their clinical years.

F.   Education of medical students, particularly in the first two years of medical school, requires substantial experience in fundamental science (e.g. anatomy, genetics, pathology, etc). This requires large and small classrooms as well as various kinds of laboratories for instruction. As the academic health center develops, courses for medical students doing their first two years could be provided by a combination of teachers in the research institute, scientists at UT Austin, and well-trained physician teachers from the various affiliated teaching hospitals. Long distance learning with telecommunications connected to UTMB would provide an important component of this portion of medical student education.

G.   Seton and St. David's Hospitals currently sponsor residency training programs in internal medicine, surgery, pediatrics, psychiatry, family medicine and O8/Gyn. These programs could be transitioned to UTMB sponsorship and additional residency programs established in collaboration with Austin Hospitals. There is a significant cadre of highly-trained local clinicians, who could be recruited within the Austin area as teachers in these programs, in addition to new teachers who are recruited as part of faculty research programs.

H.   The School of Public Health (SPH) at The University of Texas Health Science Center at Houston is currently developing a collaboration with UT Austin for research and education including a joint MD/MPH program, Collaborations with other UT institutions such as the University of Texas Health Science Center at San Antonio, could be developed as part of the research and educational activities in Austin. Collaborations with Texas A&M already exist with the SPH and could be expanded to other educational and research programs. Programs in nursing, pharmacy and allied health education will also be facilitated.

1. Progressive expansion of educational programs, particularly those involving graduate medical education residencies would substantially contribute to the growing demand for care of indigent medical patients. Expansion of these programs would also contribute to an increased number of physicians practicing in Texas.

The development of a series of research institutes, and the recruitment of UTMB faculty who, with collaborators at UT Austin, would conduct high-quality research and participate in outstanding educational programs would allow a progressive expansion in the number of medical students and post-graduate medical residents who could be educated in Austin. This incremental approach would not require complex steps associated with accreditation of an entirely new medical school, but could be accomplished with the guidance and responsibility of UTMB. If over the course of ten to twelve years, critical mass developed and resources allowed the establishment of a complete medical school, accreditation for such a unit could be proposed as part of UTMB. In this organizational structure, the Dean of the medical school would report to the President of UTMB and have a programmatic relationship to the President of UT Austin. The governance structure of the medical school could be established, which would guarantee appropriate representation from faculty of UT Austin with that of UTMB faculty. Indeed many of these faculty members would have joint appointments.

There are several important advantages to this incremental strategy. Each step would involve the addition of quality personnel and programs in their own right, pending available resources for the next step. With the rate of increase in federal funds for biomedical research decreasing over the next few years, it is essential that Texas position itself to be highly competitive for these funds and the economic benefits and development that can be derived from research supported with these monies. A health center/UT Austin synergism would be remarkably competitive in this regard and almost certainly would be significantly more successful than could be accomplished individually.

Texas currently has 150 physicians per 100,000 population, compared to a national average of 200 physicians per 100,000 population. With continued rapid growth of the population in Texas, the increasing number of older individuals requiring medical care, and the shortage that exists at present, efforts to increase physician recruitment through expanded graduate medical programs and increasing the number of medical students will be essential.

As facilities and resources developed in Austin, progressive increases in both residents and medical students could be accomplished.

Ultimately a four-year medical school would contribute to all of these goals. Moreover, the transfer of technology from research programs and medical programs which would evolve from this *effort* would have critical additional economic benefit to Austin and Texas.

Hypothetical Work plan:

The following approach to developing an academic health center in Austin is absolutely dependent upon the availability of funds at each step. The incremental approach has the advantage that steps are taken as funds become available, and the resulting investment can stand on its own until the next steps are taken.

2004 to 2006

Obtain a site for development of an academic health center, for example, the former Mueller Airport.

Obtain funding for a research institute (for example neurosciences/cardiovascular/cancer genetics) requiring resources primarily from private donors. TRB funding could be requested for building construction, but a successful institute would require a large endowment for operations and recruitment of a world-class faculty, The facility would include some clinical and classroom space.

Additional residency training programs will be established and expanded in Austin hospitals under the direction of UTMB, in internal medicine, pediatrics, family medicine and emergency medicine.

Obtain branch campus status for UTMB with an increase of its class size to 225 and additional legislative funding.

Medical students from both the third and fourth year classes at UTMB would continue to participate in clerkships in Austin hospitals. Currently 23 students spend the entire third year in Austin and 50-60 participate in fourth year clerkships. Recruitment of additional clinical faculty for expanded residency programs and in anticipation of more medical students would be increased.

As soon as a clear financial commitment to the research institute is identified, the search for a national director would be undertaken. Construction of the first research institute would be begun.

<u>2006 to 2009</u>

The Central Texas Veterans Administration would open an inpatient and ambulatory clinic at the Mueller site with enhanced opportunities for resident and medical student training and research collaborations. Students would be recruited for the MD/PhD program, jointly run by UTMB and UT Austin. 8 to 12 students would be matriculated each year.

Recruitment would commence for a high-quality faculty for the first research institute whose construction would be completed in this time-frame. Additional clinical faculty would be recruited who are involved in the translation of science to clinical application in the research institute.

Additional residency positions would be developed in general surgery, surgical specialties and dermatology within affiliated primary teaching hospitals.

<u>2007 to 2008</u>

Funding for a second research institute would be provided primarily from private sources.

<u>2008 to 2010</u>

A director and faculty for the second institute would be recruited.

<u>2010 to 2012</u>

The number of UTMB medical students rotating through the third and fourth year would increase to 60 in the third year and 75-80 in the fourth year. Basic science courses for medical students in their first two years and for MD/PhD students would be conducted in Austin through a combination of UT Austin faculty, faculty at the research institutes and distance learning from UTMB. Additional funding would be obtained for an expanded instruction, including classrooms for small group instruction, auditoria and learning laboratories. These facilities would provide classroom space for an incoming medical school class of 75 to 80 students per year.

2014

The first class would be admitted to the Austin medical school. The dean of the medical school would report directly to the president of UTMB with a programmatic relationship in reporting to the president of UT Austin. The governance of the school would be established in such a way that there was formal and continuing involvement of leadership from UT Austin in the program of the medical school, although operations would be the responsibility of UTMB. The initial class might be in the range of 100 to 125 students, although in subsequent years this could increase significantly.

Under this approach the research enterprise would depend heavily on private funding. However, the Legislature could consider authorizing tuition revenue bonds for the construction of the research and instructional space. As the opportunities develop for increasing the absolute number of medical students through the UTMB/Austin program, additional funding would be requested through the application of formula funding. Depending on the financial condition of the state, the legislature may choose to provide resources for infrastructure and operations.

APPENDIX 5

Board of Regents Minutes, "Proposed Austin Academic Health Center," August 11, 2004

6.   U. T. System: Proposed Austin Academic Health Center

REPORT

Dr. Kenneth Shine, Executive Vice Chancellor for Health Affairs will present an overview of interest and opportunities for the development of an academic health Center in Austin.

Considerable opportunities exist for the expansion of biomedical research, education, and training programs in Austin. The University of Texas at Austin, a major research institution, would benefit significantly from interactions with biomedical scientists and health researchers. Such research activities could translate into further economic development.

Expansion of educational opportunities for medical students and training for resident physicians would enhance health and healthcare in general, and particularly provide care for the medically indigent in the community. Research and training programs would also attract outstanding faculty physicians who would contribute to healthcare and would add to the attractiveness of the city to employers, employees, and their families.

The U. T. Medical Branch–Galveston has a long history of academic affiliations in Austin. Twenty-three medical students spend their third year training in Austin hospitals. Many other students take electives in Austin so that at any given time as many as 100 medical students are present. A new women's health hospital was opened under the direction of U. T. Medical Branch–Galveston at the Seton/Brackenridge Hospital. This program has received approval for a resident physician training program in obstetrics and gynecology. A state-of-the-art, fast MRI, imaging program is now under joint development by the U. T. Medical Branch–Galveston, U. T. Austin and the Central Texas Veterans Administration. U. T. Medical Branch–Galveston and U. T. Austin are now organizing a joint M.D./Ph.D. program.

Opportunities for an academic health center in Austin include the development of a regional school of public health, created by U. T. Health Science Center–Houston in collaboration with U. T. Austin, as well as collaborations with U. T. Health Science Center–San Antonio and other health institutions.

An academic health center could be developed in Austin through a series of incremental steps which would build research, education, patient care capacity over time. Such an academic health center could be developed in accordance with the following principles:

a. Each component of the enterprise must be of the highest quality so as to recruit a world-class faculty and develop outstanding educational and clinical programs.

b. Each step would be taken only if adequate funding were available for that portion of the program. Considerable private support would be required for this purpose.

c. An incremental approach would be taken to increase the number of programs for undergraduate students seeking M.D. or M.D./Ph.D. degrees, and the addition of postgraduate residency training programs in the various medical specialties.

d. The academic health center should be physically located proximate to the U. T. Austin campus, in order to synergize the capacities of each enterprise.

e. An academic medical center would require the establishment of one or more medical research institutes which capitalize on synergies with U. T. Austin. An institute might focus on developmental biology, neurosciences, systems biology, cancer genetics or other aspects of molecular medicine. Substantial support from private donors would be required to create such an institution.

f. U. T. Medical Branch–Galveston would continue to develop educational and research programs in collaboration with the new Austin Children's Hospital, the Central Texas Veterans Administration, Seton/Brackenridge Hospital, St. David's Hospital and other clinical sites for student and residency training.

g. The School of Public Health at U. T. Health Science Center–Houston would continue to develop collaborations with U. T. Austin for research and education.

\

h.   Other institutions including U. T. San Antonio, U. T. Health Science Center -Houston, and Texas A&M University would be encouraged to enter into collaborations in medicine, nursing, pharmacy, allied health and other areas.

The development of expanded educational programs, including residencies, would contribute substantially to the provision of care for the medically indigent individuals. It would also contribute to an increased number of physicians practicing in Texas.

In a time of profound fiscal constraints in the State, development of these academic health programs would require substantial public and private partnerships in which the local community and local donors would have to provide substantial resources for the development of an academic health center.

While there have been no negotiations with the City of Austin, it has been reported that the City of Austin proposes to set aside 15 acres on the former Mueller Airport site for medical purposes. This site is proximate to the new Children's Hospital. A more fully developed academic health center would require substantially more space. However this property might form the initial location of the educational, research, or clinical facilities essential to developing an Academic Health Center.

Considerable public interest has been expressed in Austin to create a medical school in the community. It is possible that the incremental developments described above might lead, at some future time, to formal establishment of such a school. However incremental and gradual expansion of programs by U. T. Medical Branch–Galveston an already fully accredited institution, could continue, without the immediate major financial resources required for a new medical school. Incremental development of research program offers opportunities to recruit a small core of world class scientists upon which a great faculty could be built. This development will require effective public-private synergies and resources for its accomplishment. There does seem to be a convergence of interest and opportunity upon which to build.

Organization and Governance, Academic Health Center

ORGANIZATION AND GOVERNANCE

The creation of an Academic Health Center in Austin will be facilitated by its development in collaboration with a mature academic health center. Overall leadership will be provided by President John Stobo of The University of Texas Medical Branch at Galveston (UTMB). The Deans of each professional school report to Dr. Stobo. These include schools of medicine, nursing, allied health and graduate studies.

Medical education in Austin is under the direction of the Regional Dean for Medical education, Dr. Thomas Blackwell. He is responsible for the operations of the education program for medical students and Graduate Medical Education. Appendix F describes the five-year plan for Graduate Medical Education, which is currently being implemented. UTMB and the Seton Health System have signed a long term (up to 30 years) agreement for the further development of medical education in central Texas. Dr. Blackwell is also responsible for coordination of educational activities with Veterans Administration Clinical Programs.

Initially the Academic Health Center would include the Children's Health Research Institute. This institute and an additional two institutes to be developed on the Academic Health Campus, would be headed by a Scientific Director who reports administratively to the president of UTMB, with a close programmatic responsibility to the president of The University of Texas at Austin (UT Austin). The Director would be advised by a scientific advisory committee including faculty members from UTMB and UT Austin. There would also be a Director's Council which will include community representatives. The Director will be responsible for overall management of the institute including equipment, program development and resource development.

Faculty will have joint appointments at UT Austin and UTMB with their primary appointment based upon their area of expertise and professional interests. It is likely that basic scientists will have primary appointments at UT Austin, with a secondary appointment at UTMB, while clinical investigators will have their primary appointment at UTMB and a secondary appointment at UT Austin.

Upon completion of administrative buildings and classrooms, a Medical School Dean and Vice President for the Austin Academic Health Center enterprise will be appointed. At that time the Institute's Director will report to the Academic Health Center Dean and Vice President. Overall responsibility for the effort resides with the University of Texas Board System of Regents.

Robert Mueller Municipal Airport Plan Implementation Advisory Commission, 2004–2005 Members

2004–2005 CURRENT MEMBERS
ROBERT MUELLER MUNICIPAL AIRPORT (RMMA) PLAN
IMPLEMENTATION ADVISORY COMMISSION

Donna Carter/Orban Design

Rick Krivoniak/Member at Large

Matt Harris/Neighborhood

Larry McKee/Neighborhood

Tracy Dour Atkins/Business Position

Jim Walker/Neighborhood

Jim Robertson/Architecture

Rob Carruthers/Commercial

CITY OF AUSTIN STAFF

Office of Economic Growth and Redevelopment Services

One Texas Center, Suite 1300

505 Barton Springs Road

P. O. Box 1088

Main Office: 974-7819

Pamela Hefner, ASLA

Principal Planner

9/21/04

[contact information redacted]

UT Austin / UTMB Collaboration, August 24, 2004

AUSTIN ACADEMIC HEALTH CENTER
UT AUSTIN/UTMB COLLABORATION

The student enrollment in Austin was to be undertaken as part of the accreditation of the UT Medical Branch. Although some Coordinating Board approvals may be required for increasing class sizes, no authorization for new programs would be required. The campus could be separately accredited when fully developed.

This approach was based on the gradual expansion of medical student programs in Austin accompanied by the construction of research facilities, and new recruitment of a basic science faculty who would teach the first two years of medical school. At the same time clinical programs would be developed in relation to the Seton Health System, staffed primarily by physicians in practice at these facilities, many of whom are graduates of UTMB. Superspecialists would be recruited in specific relationship to research programs. For example, if the first research program were a children's health research institute, pediatricians would be recruited to participate in translational research that would ultimately become involved in medical school education as well.

Medical school enrollment would be progressively increased with the permission of the Coordinating Board and Liaison Committee on Medical Education, but no new program would be required over the first five to eight years. This will allow the availability of formula funding to underwrite cost of the expanded program as the number of students is increased incrementally. According to this plan three research facilities would be built over a period of six to nine years on the Mueller Airport site. In the first two to three years, a clinic facility would be constructed by the Veteran's Administration on the same site. In the third year of the program a combination of permanent university funds and tuition revenue bonds would be used to erect the first classroom and lecture hall building. In subsequent years an administration building, library and allied health center would be constructed. An opportunity for a fourth research building as part of Stage Two is also feasible.

According to this plan the initial construction expenditures would be approximately $710 million, with the first $650 million funded through indirect returns from progressive staffing at the Mueller research facilities. $30–50 million would be available for recruiting of basic scientists for these research facilities from overall operating costs are included in the financing package. Because of the availability of infrastructure support such as facilities and construction, contracts and grants, student services, medical billing services, etc., provided by UTMB there would be little incremental facilities costs. Construction of two additional medical school buildings could take place anytime from the ninth to twelfth year of the venture with funding from tuition revenue bonds and philanthropy. Incremental addition of medical students would allow for progressive increases in monies for operating costs under this plan.

Over the next several years residencies programs will be expanded in medicine, surgery, pediatrics, obstetrics, gynecology, and other subspecialties under an affiliation agreement between UTMB and Seton Health System. UTMB would continue collaborative projects with the UT Austin campus, continue their imaging center MD/PhD programs, etc. UTMB would continue to operate Women's Hospital at Brackenridge Hospital and collaborate with the Veteran's Administration in operation on the to be constructed VA Clinic Facility.

Overview and Update: An Academic Health Center in Austin, July 14, 2005

OVERVIEW AND UPDATE: AN ACADEMIC HEALTH CENTER IN AUSTIN WITH THE UNIVERSITY OF TEXAS MEDICAL BRANCH AND ITS PARTNERS

July 14, 2005

Austin is a rapidly growing metropolitan area: the current five-county area population of 1.5 million is expected to top 2 million in the next 20 years (Office of the State Demographer, State of Texas). According to the Texas State Board of Medical Examiners, the Austin area will encounter corresponding physician shortages as the population increases. Austin is the largest city in the US without a medical school or academic medical center. Nevertheless, The University of Texas Medical Branch at Galveston has had a long relationship with Austin's Brackenridge Hospital, both in medical student and resident education. Brackenridge is the oldest public hospital in Texas, established in 1884, and UTMB-Galveston, established in 1891, was the state's first medical school and teaching hospital. Brackenridge has participated in medical education since 1931. The partnership between UTMB with Brackenridge is a "natural".

In 1972, the Travis County Medical Society founded the Central Texas Medical Foundation (CTMF) to sponsor graduate medical education programs at Brackenridge Hospital and to employ full-time salaried faculty for its programs. CTMF sponsors residencies in Internal Medicine, Pediatrics, Family Medicine, Psychiatry, and the transitional year; CTMF and Brackenridge has participated in integrated programs in OB-Gyn and Surgery in collaboration with St. Joseph's

Hospital in Houston. In 1996, Seton HealthCare Network contracted with the City of Austin to operate Brackenridge and Children's Hospital and in the process acquired CTMF. In 2000, CTMF assumed the name Austin Medical Education Program (AMEP). In 2004, UTMB contracted with the City of Austin and Seton to operate the Austin Women's Hospital within Brackenridge Hospital. Seton is constructing a major Children's Medical Center at the site of the former Mueller airport (about 1-½ miles from Brackenridge), to be completed in 2007.

In the last three years, the concept of a UTMB-Galveston regional campus in Austin evolved, and a strategic planning group, Central Texas Institute for Research & Education in Medicine & Biotechnology (CTI), was formed. This organization includes UTMB, Seton HealthCare Network, St. David's HealthCare Partnership, the Central Texas Veterans Health Care System, UT Austin, the UT Health Science Center at Houston's School of Public Health, and the Greater Austin Chamber of Commerce. CTI's major goal is to create an academic health campus in Austin (See www.cti-med.org for more about the organization and its vision and goals).

CTI's vision is based on a desire to capitalize on the breadth and depth of health related education and research at UT Austin. The group has: reached consensus on the regional campus concept; begun specific planning to realize the concept; briefed the UT System Board of Regents, the Legislature, community leaders, and potential donors; and begun to identify space and funding for academic facilities. UTMB has been offered 27 acres at the Mueller airport site, adjacent to the new Children's Center, for construction of research institutes and academic buildings.

These negotiations are underway by the UT System, but a decision has not been made regarding the site for the academic health campus.

UTMB has developed and implemented formal undergraduate medical education, which now places 23 junior medical students in Austin, with the same curriculum as in Galveston. Measures of success on educational testing and ability to achieve their desired residencies have indicated no difference between students educated in Austin or Galveston. A large number of UTMB fourth-year students spend time in Austin on electives with similar success. An infrastructure has developed, and UTMB is rapidly moving to place up to 50 students in Austin for the entire third and fourth years. Their curricular needs have resulted in plans for additional GME programs sponsored by UTMB and located in Austin.

A new UTMB OB-Gyn residency program was accredited in 2004 and has successfully recruited its first class through NRMP for July 2005. Current plans are to transfer the sponsorship of the Internal Medicine, Pediatrics, Family Medicine, Psychiatry, and Transitional year programs from AMEP to UTMB within the next 18–24 months. UTMB, in partnership with Seton/Brackenridge, the Central Texas VA, and practicing neurologists and neuroscientists in Austin, has applied for accreditation for a neurology residency program. This program takes advantage of the great neuroscience strengths in Austin: academically-oriented clinicians and practitioners; faculty and investigators at UT Austin; the resources of the Seton HealthCare Network, Brackenridge Hospital, and the Central Texas Veterans Health Care System; and the AMEP faculty. UT Austin and the Central Texas VA are jointly constructing a facility for a research brain-imaging center, in which UTMB will have a major role.

UTMB and Seton/Brackenridge are now planning and will seek accreditation of a Surgery residency. Plans are also being discussed to develop training programs in hematology/oncology and gastroenterology.

UTMB and UT Austin presently have joint MD/PhD programs in neuroscience, bioengineering, and molecular biology; others are planned. Together, all of these resources provide a broad and highly competent base upon which to build undergraduate medical education, graduate medical education, and research.

The mutual vision of UTMB and its partners continues to be to create a world-class academic research and education center in Austin.

Board of Regents Minutes, January 12, 2006

SPECIAL ITEM

U. T. SYSTEM: FOLLOW-UP REPORT ON
AUSTIN ACADEMIC HEALTH CENTER

Executive Vice Chancellor Shine presented an update on a potential Academic Health Center In Austin as discussed with the Board at the August 11, 2004 meeting.

Dr. Mary Ann Rankin, Dean of the College of Natural Sciences at The University of Texas at Austin, spoke and there was discussion. Chairman Huffines asked that a presentation on the proposed Austin Academic Health Center and financial data be scheduled for a future Board meeting.

RECESS TO EXECUTIVE SESSION.—At 2:55 p.m., Chairman Huffines announced the Board would recess to convene in Executive Session pursuant to Texas Government Code Sections 551.071, 551.072, 551.073, and 551.074 to consider those matters listed on the Executive Session agenda.

RECONVENE IN OPEN SESSION.—At 4:15 p.m., the Board reconvened in open session and took the following action on matters discussed in Executive Session.

1. U. T. System and U. T. Austin: Potential negotiated gift involving a naming opportunity

    No action was taken on a potential negotiated gift involving a naming opportunity at The University of Texas System and The University of Texas at Austin.

2. U. T. Pan American: Discussion and appropriate action on pending litigation titled Board of Regents of The University of Texas System v. Geraldine F. Glick and Robert Edward Glick, Joint Independent Executors of the Estate of Kenith S. Glick, Deceased: Martha P. Glick and Judith Gall Glick, Joint Independent Executors of the Estate of Kemper H. Glick, Deceased: Geraldine F. Glick, Individually: Martha P. Glick, Individually: and Gordon Bloomfield regarding the purchase of approximately 18.96 acres of land with improvements out of Lot 4, Block 273, Texas-Mexican Railway Company's Survey, in Edinburg, Hidalgo County, Texas; for parking and for campus expansion

Regent McHugh moved that the U. T. System Board of Regents

a. reaffirm the authorization to the Executive Director of Real Estate to acquire on behalf of The University of Texas–Pan American

AGENDA ITEM 2

U. T. SYSTEM: FOLLOW-UP REPORT ON AUSTIN
ACADEMIC HEALTH CENTER

REPORT

Executive Vice Chancellor Shine will present an update on a potential Academic Health Center in Austin as discussed with the Board at the August 11, 2004 meeting. During the 2004 meeting, Dr. Shine made a report entitled Proposed Austin Academic Health Center; a copy is attached on Pages 34–34b. Materials Dr. Shine will use during his presentation are set forth on Pages 34c–34g.

Note: See appendix 6 for the 2004 report.

Board of Regents Presentation, January 12, 2006

Presentation to the Board
of Regents
January 12, 2006

Austin Academic Health
Center

Austin Academic Health Center

- Medical Education
- Biomedical Research
- Nursing
- Pharmacy
- Public Health (Houston)
- Health Care

Principles

- Highest Quality
- Incremental Approach
- Adequate Funding at Each Step
- Considerable Private Support
- Proximate to UT Austin (Mueller Site?)
- Partnership of UT Austin and UT Health Science Schools

3

Mueller Site

- Catellus (Developer)
- 15 Acres Long Term Lease (Nominal Cost)
- 12 Acres Purchase/Option (City Council Approval)
- Research Buildings (4)
- VA Clinic?
- Educational Buildings
- Proximate to Children's Hospital

4

Mueller Site

- Good Neighbors
- Compatible Design Features
- Retail/?Children's Museum
- No Further Expansion on Site

5

Educational/Clinical Programs - UTMB

- Women's Hospital
- OB/GYN Residency
- Seton System/UTMB Affiliation Agreement
- Medical Students (~120)
- Imaging Center (Joint UTMB/VA/Austin)
- MD/PhD Program/Austin
- Community Clinics
- Cancer Program/Brackenridge

6

Biomedical Research

- UT Austin/Dean Mary Ann Rankin
  - Programs/Appointments
- Biomedical Research Institutes/Translational
- Children's Health Research Institute
  - Developmental Biology
  - Genetics
  - Nutrition
- Neurosciences
- Heart Disease/Cancer

7

Community Support

- Continued Strong Broad-Based Interest
- Offers to Help
- Economic Development
- Recruiting Executives
- Community Health Needs

8

Next Steps

- Continue Clinical/Educational Programs
- Continue UT Austin Collaborations with Health Campuses
- Pursue Philanthropic Opportunities Focused Upon Biomedical Research Institute(s) Especially Children's Health Research

9

Austin Academic Health Center Children's Health Research Institute Report

Austin Academic Health Center
ᐧChildren's Health Research Institute

Interest continues to grow in the creation of an academic health center in Austin. When appropriate, the University of Texas Medical Branch (UTMB) is committed to expanding educational opportunities for medical students and residents. At the present time approximately 100 UTMB medical students are learning in Austin each year, an OB/GYN residency program has recently been accredited at the Austin Women's Hospital and further expansion of residency programs may occur over the next several years.

UTMB has launched a research program in medical imaging in Austin, in collaboration with the Veterans Administration and the University of Texas at Austin (UT Austin). This facility will be located at the Pickle Research Campus in North Austin. An MD/PhD program is currently being developed between UTMB a'1d UT Austin to train young medical scientists. In patient care, UTMB operates the Austin Women's Hospital at Brackenridge.

The School of Public Health at UT Health Science Center at Houston is currently in conversation with UT Austin to develop a program in public health. UT Austin has a School of Nursing which ranks 7th in the United States for research funding and a superb School of Pharmacy. However the opportunity to capitalize on research development at UT Austin is limited for health related discoveries in the absence of strong biomedical research and clinical trial programs in Austin. President Larry Faulkner of UT Austin has publicly stated his belief that the development of an academic health center in Austin would be of great value to the university campus.

Establishment of an academic health campus largely as the responsibility of the UTMB has great advantages. These include the opportunity to expand medical education and teaching programs without the difficult challenge of accreditation of a brand new medical school. Even if such a school were to ultimately achieve independent status, this would be far easier at a time when there is a critical mass of faculty and programs. The Veterans Administration has expressed significant interest in the creation of a clinical facility to provide ambulatory care for veterans in Austin. This would provide additional opportunities for clinical research and education.

However, the recruitment of a world-class clinical faculty to Austin will require the development of serious research programs so that the faculty recruited can believe that they are part of a world-class, cutting-age enterprise, which translates newest developments in research to the care of patients. For this reason, the creation of a children's research institute by The University of Texas

1

System (UT System) would be the initial step to galvanize the development of an academic health center in Austin. The Children's Health Institute would be created as a world-class center for fundamental science and clinical research for the benefit of children's health. It would be organized around the concept of a translational center, that is of expeditiously applying the latest results in science to the care of patients through a rapid translational process. Such an activity requires basic scientists, clinical scientists, experts in human clinical trials, clinicians, epidemiologists, pediatricians and other health professionals.

An essential part of the translational process is the interaction between clinician and scientist. Interaction is a two-way iterative process in which problems identified in the clinic can be studied, hypotheses developed in the laboratory and evaluated in patients.

The creation of a children's health institute in Austin would have numerous benefits:

1. New laboratory studies of critical issues in children's health could be undertaken in close collaboration with the faculty at UT Austin. Mary Ann Rankin, Dean of Natural Sciences at UT Austin, emphasizes the institution's commitment to developmental biology. And UTMB has several programs centered around health issues of women and children.

2. The creation of a world-class scientific environment would attract outstanding clinicians who would conduct clinical trials as well as interact in the scientific activities of the basic sciences. These pediatricians would also be available to enrich clinical care in the Austin area.

3. The close proximity of the new Dell Children's Medical Center provides an opportunity for translational research to occur. In addition the identification of the children's health research institute as a world-class site for dealing with difficult disorders in children would be attractive to patients who might come to the Dell Children's Medical Center from considerable distances.

4. Such a program would synergize well with the commitment of UTMB to women's health in the Austin Women's Hospital where prenatal diagnosis, the influence of the fetal environment on development and the discovery of interventions that would promote the birth of a healthy fetus would be a great advance. Moreover, such research activities would have a direct effect to improve the health of mothers.

The translational interactions of the children's health research institute may include the following components:

2

A.
1. The genetic and molecular basis of normal and abnormal child development
2. The environmental factors interacting with genetics to alter normal and abnormal child development
3. Maternal factors occurring during pregnancy which affect development
4. The fundamental aspects of normal and abnormal psychological development in children
5. Genetic and environmental factors affecting learning and learning disorders

B. Clinical Trials Program. This component would assess the effectiveness and risks of genetic treatments, biological agents, drugs and behavioral interventions designed to guide the healthy development of children.

C. Pediatric care programs in which infants and children (as well as pregnant mothers) would be seen for the study of complex and perplexing disorders. Patients seen in these clinics would receive the best available treatment and would also be offered opportunities in research protocols developed as a consequence of institute research.

Other important components of the institute would include expertise in technology transfer and new product development, bioethics related to both research and treatment, and educational outreach programs conducted in collaboration with the Dell Children's Medical Center around discoveries made in the institute. .

Success of the institute would require recruitment of a world-class scientist as Director and a number of other important investigators. Those recruited to the institute would have their academic appointments at UT Austin and UT Medical Branch.

The institute would be fiscally managed by UTMB. Its director would report to the President of UTMB for fiscal issues, but would report to the President of UT Austin and UTMB for programmatic oversight. A scientific advisory committee composed of faculty from both UT Austin and UTMB would serve to advise the director, in addition to an extramural advisory committee of scientists outside of the two institutions.

A community advisory committee would also serve in support of the enterprise.

It is anticipated that the institute would operate in a building of 150,000 gross square feet, preferably on a site adjacent to the Dell Children's Medical Center. The estimated cost for 5 years in successfully developing a world-class enterprise would be approximately $175 million dollars (see attached appendix

3

1). The plans for this institute are consistent with the presentation made to the UT System Board of Regents on August 30, 2004 (see appendix 2).

4

Board of Regents Minutes, Dell Pediatric Research Institute, August 10, 2006

3. **U. T. Austin: Dell Pediatric Research Institute—Request for approval of design development; approval of evaluation of alternative energy economic feasibility; appropriation of funds and authorization of expenditure; and resolution regarding parity debt**

RECOMMENDATION

The Chancellor concurs with the Interim Executive Vice Chancellor for Academic Affairs, the Executive Vice Chancellor for Business Affairs, and President Powers that the U. T. System Board of Regents approve the recommendations for the Dell Pediatric Research Institute project at The University of Texas at Austin as follows:

Project No: 102-257
Project Delivery Method: Design/Build
Substantial Completion Date: November 2008

Total Project Cost:	*Source*	*Current*
	Gifts	$38,000,000
	Grants	$38,000,000
	Revenue Financing System Bond Proceeds	$21,000,000
		$97,000,000

a. approve design development plans;
b. approval of evaluation of alternative energy economic feasibility;
c. appropriate funds and authorize expenditure of funds; and

d. resolve in accordance with Section 5 of the Amended and Restated Master Resolution Establishing The University of Texas System Revenue Financing System that

- parity debt shall be issued to pay the project's cost, including any costs prior to the issuance of such parity debt;

- sufficient funds will be available to meet the financial obligations of the U. T. System, including sufficient Pledged Revenues as defined in the Master Resolution to satisfy the Annual Debt Service Requirements of the Financing System, and to meet all financial obligations of the U. T. System Board of Regents relating to the Financing System; and

- U. T. Austin, which is a "Member" as such term is used in the Master Resolution, possesses the financial capacity to satisfy its direct obligation as defined in the Master Resolution relating to the issuance by the U. T. System Board of Regents of tax-exempt parity debt in the aggregate amount of $21,000,000.

BACKGROUND INFORMATION

DEBT SERVICE

The $21,000,000 in Revenue Financing System debt will be repaid from indirect cost recovery resulting from new research activity at the Dell Pediatric Research Institute as well as parking and retail revenues attributable to the garage and stores. Average annual debt service on the project is estimated at $1.53 million. Once fully occupied, the project's debt service coverage ratio is expected to be at least 2.9 times.

PREVIOUS BOARD ACTION

On June 20, 2006, the project was included in the Capital Improvement Program (CIP) with a preliminary project cost of $97,000,000 with funding of $38,000,000 from Gifts, $38,000,000 from Grants, and $21,000,000 from Revenue Financing System Bond Proceeds.

PROJECT DESCRIPTION

This project will establish a pediatric health research institute in Austin. Combining U. T. Austin's core expertise in life sciences with the new Dell Children's Medical Center will establish Austin as a center of excellence for children's health and biomedical research.

The Dell Pediatric Research Institute is to be constructed on the former Robert Mueller Airport site, adjacent to the new Dell Children's Medical Center of Central Texas. It is anticipated the Dell Pediatric Research Institute will comply with the guidelines of the Master Plan established for the development of the former Robert Mueller Airport site. U. T. Austin will provide funding if gift funding is not available.

BASIS OF DESIGN

The planned building life expectancy includes the following elements:

- Enclosure: 25–40 years
- Building Systems: 15–20 years
- Interior Construction: 10–20 years

The exterior appearance and finish will be consistent with high-end commercial research facilities. This facility is the first University of Texas building in the Mueller Master Redevelopment, and will comply with Mueller Design Guidelines.

The mechanical and electrical building systems will be designed with sufficient flexibility and space for future capacity to allow for programmatic changes without significant disruption to ongoing research.

The interior appearance and finish will include open, flexible, generic lab space with central lab utilities and support space.

Texas Government Code Section 2166.403 requires the governing body of a State agency to verify in an open meeting the economic feasibility of incorporating alternative energy devices into a new State building or an addition to an existing building. Therefore, the Project Architect prepared a renewable energy evaluation for this project in accordance with the Energy Conservation Design Standards for New State Buildings. This evaluation determined that alternative energy devices such as solar, wind, biomass, or photovoltaic energy are not economically feasible for the project.

The economic impact of the project was reported to the U. T. System Board of Regents as part of the design development presentation.

APPENDIX 14

Dell Pediatric Research Institute Executive Summary Report, UT System Office of Facilities, Planning, and Construction

THE UNIVERSITY *of* TEXAS SYSTEM
FOURTEEN INSTITUTIONS. UNLIMITED POSSIBILITIES.

102-257 The Dell Pediatric Research Institute
The University of Texas at Austin

Executive Summary Report

Project Description

The Dell Pediatric Research Institute, The University of Texas at Austin project follows a generous gift from the Michael and Susan Dell Foundation to the university. The project will be the first institution designed for The University of Texas Health Research Campus within the redevelopment of the former Robert Mueller Municipal Airport. The 150,000 GSF high-end commercial laboratory building will be designed to be flexible with both wet and dry (computational) research labs and with a 1:1 ratio of open bench laboratory space to hard-wall laboratory support space. Appropriate office space, including a suite for the Director and staff, and necessary building support space will be included in the design. The building will accommodate a minimum of 28 Principal Investigators, each with a staff of 10 including senior technicians, post-doctoral scientists, and graduate students. In addition, a ~30,000 GSF vivarium will be included to support the research within this building and in future build

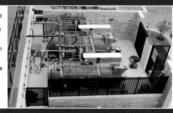

Project Information

Project Status:	Complete
Project Delivery Method:	Design/Build
CIP Project Type:	New
Gross and Assignable Square Feet:	GSF: 149,653 ASF: 89,792
Phase and Estimated % Complete:	Complete - 100%
Project Team:	Rawski, , Westmoreland, Westmoreland, Connolly
Project Advocate(s):	
Architecture Firm:	
Construction Firm:	Hensel Phelps / HOK

Project Budget

Construction Services:	$	64,286,618	at $	430 / GSF
Total Project Cost:	$	88,500,000	at $	591 / GSF

Project Funding

Gifts	$	2,500,000
Grants	$	8,000,000
Permanent University Fund Bonds	$	25,000,000
Revenue Financing System Bonds	$	53,000,000

Project Schedule

BOR/Chancellor DD Approval	08/09/2006
Issue NTP - Construction	11/06/2006
Achieve Substantial Completion	12/05/2008
Achieve Operational Occupancy	10/28/2010

Project Remarks

Close out project and transfer the balance to institution

Board Approvals

None

Board of Regents, Dell Medical School Planning Committees, July 16, 2013

STEERING COMMITTEE

CHAIR:

Steve Leslie   Executive Vice President and Provost, UT Austin

CO-CHAIRS:

Sue Cox   UTSW Regional Dean, Austin Programs

Bob Messing   Vice Provost for Biomedical Sciences Professor, College of Pharmacy, UT Austin

MEMBERS:

Trish Young Brown	President and CEO, Central Health
Lynn Crismon	Dean, College of Pharmacy, UT Austin
Greg Fenves	Dean, Cockrell School of Engineering, UT Austin
Greg Fitz	UTSW Executive VP of Academic Affairs & Provost Dean, Southwestern Medical School
Tom Gilligan	Dean, McCombs School of Business, UT Austin
Linda Hicke	Dean, College of Natural Sciences, UT Austin
Tim LaFrey	Senior VP, Seton Ventures & Alliances
Jim Lindsey	Chief Medical Officer, Seton Healthcare Family
Alexa Stuifbergen	Dean of Nursing, UT Austin
Luis Zayas	Dean of Social Work, UT Austin

ADVISORS:

Pat Clubb	Vice President for University Operations, UT Austin
Robert Cullick	Media Outreach, UT Austin
Tara Doolittle	Director of Media Outreach, UT Austin
Gwen Grigsby	Associate VP for Governmental Relations, UT Austin
Sandy Guzman	Legislative Director, Texas State Senator Kirk Watson
Kevin Hegarty	Vice President and Chief Financial Officer, UT Austin
Mike Kerker	Associate Vice Provost, UT Austin
David Laude	Senior Vice Provost for Enrollment and Graduation Management, UT Austin
Carlos Martinez	Associate Vice President for Governmental Relations, UT Austin
Pedro Reyes	Executive Vice Chancellor for Academic Affairs, UT System
Dan Slesnick	Senior Vice Provost for Resource Management, UT Austin
Gary Susswein	Director of University Media Relations, UT Austin
Amy Thomas	Vice Chancellor and Counsel for Health Affairs, UT System

SPACE/FACILITIES/INNOVATION PARK WORKING GROUP

- Pat Clubb **Co-Chair** (Vice President for University Operations, UT Austin)
- Bob Messing **Co-Chair** (Vice Provost for Biomedical Sciences, Professor, College of Pharmacy, UT Austin)
- Linda Hicke (Dean College of Natural Sciences, UT Austin)
- Sandy Guzman (Legislative Director, Texas State Senator Kirk Watson)
- Jim Lindsey (Chief Medical Officer, Seton Healthcare Family)
- Peter Rieck (VP-Facilities & Support Services, Seton Healthcare Family)
- Glen Otto (ARC)
- Dan Slesnick (Senior Vice Provost for Resource Management, UT Austin)
- Steve Warach (Executive Director, Seton/UTSW Research Institute)
- Sue Cox (UTSW Regional Dean, Austin Programs)
- Russ Poldrack (Professor of Psychology and Neurobiology and Director of the Imaging Research Center)
- Steven Kraal (Associate Vice President of Campus Planning & Facilities)

CHARGES

Guide the master planning process to choose sit design and maximize connectivity between buildings (Medical School, University Hospital, Medical Office Building, and Research Building).

Provide input to architects on preclinical, clinical, and continuing medical education programs to plan facilities for medical education in the Medical School building. This requires input from the curriculum working groups.

Guide the design of the research building to ensure appropriate space needs for labs, basic science core facilities, animal research, and administrative and IT support.

Assess desired and existing facilities at UT and Seton for clinical research and provide input for new research facilities within the medical office building and the hospital.

Work towards agreements needed to secure property for the Innovation Park and future additional space for future expansion.

Plan for expanded IT and administrative infrastructure to adhere to HIPAA standards and support expansion in basic and clinical research (expanded IACUC and IRB).

CURRICULUM WORKING GROUPS
- Sue Cox—**Co-Chair** (UTSW Regional Dean, Austin Programs)
- Lynn Crismon—**Co-Chair** (Dean, College of Pharmacy, UT Austin)
- Bob Messing (Vice Provost for Biomedical Sciences, Professor, College of Pharmacy, UT Austin)
- David Laude (Senior Vice Provost for Enrollment and Graduation Management, UT Austin)
- Jim Lindsey (Chief Medical Officer, Seton Healthcare Family)

CHARGES
Provide recommendations to the Dean regarding the four-year curriculum including longitudinal curriculum themes, capstone courses, and new technologies. Establish minimum competencies expected for all graduates of the Dell Medical School.

NEW INSTRUCTIONAL METHODS
MEMBERSHIP
- Sue Cox—**Chair** (UTSW Regional Dean, Austin Programs)
- Michael Sacks (Biomedical Engineering)
- Sacha Kopp (College of Natural Sciences)
- Gretchen Ritter (Executive Vice President & Provost, Department of Government, UT Austin)
- Pat Davis (Senior Associate Dean, College of Pharmacy, UT Austin)

- John Kappelman (Professor of Anthropology, UT Austin)
- Harrison Keller (Vice Provost for Higher Education Policy & Research, UT Austin)
- David Laude (Senior Vice Provost for Enrollment and Graduation Management, UT Austin)
- Melissa Wetzel (Assistant Professor, Department of Curriculum & Instruction, College of Education, UT Austin)
- Brent Iverson (Chair, Department of Chemistry and Biochemistry, UT Austin)
- Sean Theriault (Associate Professor, Department of Government)
- Michael Sweet (Director of Instructional Development, Center for Teaching and Learning, UT Austin)
- Kent Ellington (Program Director, Neurology Residency Program, Seton Healthcare Family)
- Dawn Zimmaro, CTL Director of Assessment, UT Austin

CHARGES

To identify cutting edge pedagogical approaches, including uses of technology that the Dell Medical School will employ.

Describe the pedagogical, assessment, technological, instructional design, and faculty development infrastructure needed to support the implementation of the curriculum.

Identify the human, financial, and physical resources needed to support the pedagogical, assessment, technological, instructional design, and faculty development infrastructure, and the associated costs of those resources.

INTERPROFESSIONAL EDUCATION
MEMBERSHIP
- Gayle Timmerman—**Chair** (School of Nursing, UT Austin)
- Pat Davis (Senior Associate Dean, College of Pharmacy, UT Austin)
- Barbara Jones (School of Social Work, UT Austin)
- Debra Lopez (College of Pharmacy, UT Austin)
- Martita Lopez (Department of Psychology, College of Liberal Arts, UT Austin)
- John Luk (UTMB Assistant Dean, UTSW Pediatrics faculty)
- Cheryl Perry (Regional Dean, UT School of Public Health, Austin campus)
- Yvonne Van Dyke (Vice President of Nursing Education, Seton)
- David Weigle (Assistant Dean of Graduate Medical Education, UTSW)

CHARGES

To design and integrate interprofessional education teaching and practice in the 4 year curriculum

PRE-CLINICAL TRAINING
MEMBERSHIP
- Sue Cox—**Chair** (UTSW Regional Dean, Austin Programs)
- Bob Messing (Vice Provost for Biomedical Sciences, Professor, College of Pharmacy, UT Austin)
- Dan Bolnick (Section of Integrative Biology, College of Natural Sciences)
- Shelley Payne (College of Natural Sciences)
- Kristen Harris (Section of Neurobiology, College of Natural Sciences)
- Lauren Myers (Division of Statistics and Scientific Computation, College of Natural Sciences)
- Marc Musick (College of Liberal Arts)
- Rick Morrisett (College of Pharmacy, UT Austin)

DRAFT CHARGES

Design the pre-clinical curriculum that integrates basic and clinical biomedical sciences into the first two years of the curriculum.

Design evaluation tools and appraisal instruments used to monitor student progress through the curriculum.

Ensure that the planned curriculum and evaluation instruments meet requirements for Liaison Committee on Medical Education accreditation.

> Plan to add a sub working group for **Capstone Programs and Longitudinal themes**—for example a working group to design the Art of being a Physician Course. This longitudinal course introduces and develops the students' history taking and physical diagnosis skills. Additionally, this course incorporates topics of professionalism, ethical practice, fundamentals of patient safety, inter-professional communication skills, and team work.

Longitudinal Themes (woven throughout all 4 years)
Art of being a Physician (Academic Colleges)
Ethics / Humanities
Geriatrics and Principles of Palliative Care
Culture, Health and Society
Patient Safety and Quality

Social Medicine (Ted Held and Melissa Smith)
Preventive Medicine/ Wellness

Capstone Courses: History of Medicine, Nutrition
Tracks: Research, Global Health, Public Health Policy, Biomedical Engineering

CLINICAL TRAINING

DRAFT RECOMMENDATIONS FOR MEMBERSHIP CONSIDERATION

- Nile Barnes
- Emily Doyle
- Jim Lindsey
- John Luk
- Beth Miller

DRAFT CHARGES

RESEARCH WORKING GROUP

MEMBERSHIP

- Bob Messing—**Chair** (Vice Provost for Biomedical Sciences, UT Austin)
- Steve Warach (Executive Director, Seton/UTSW Research Institute)
- Marc Musick (College of Liberal Arts)
- Dean Appling (College of Natural Sciences, Associate Dean for Research, UT Austin)
- John Ekerdt (Cockrell School of Engineering associate dean for research, UT Austin)
- Dan Johnston (Director, Institute for Neuroscience)
- Tinsley Oden (Associate Vice President for Research)
- Laura Suggs (Assoc. Chair Biomedical Engineering, Cockrell School of Engineering, UT Austin)
- Cheryl Perry (Regional Dean, UT School of Public Health, Austin campus)
- Stephen Pont (UTSW faculty in Austin, community-based research)

DRAFT CHARGES

Identify opportunities for research in basic sciences, social sciences and engineering within UT Colleges, and affiliated research centers and research units.

Develop plans for MD-PhD and other joint degree programs based at UT Austin, and possible merger of existing programs that involve other UT Health Science Centers.

Develop a program for medical students to pursue research, likely during the fourth year, not necessarily leading to a combined degree.

HEALTHCARE COMMUNITY ENGAGEMENT GROUP

(10–20 health care and or bioscience industry members, primary local):

MEMBERSHIP

- Jim Lindsey—**Chair** (Seton Healthcare Family)
- Mary Lou Adams (UT-Austin Family Nurse Practitioner Program)
- Reginald Baptiste (Cardiothoracic Surgery)
- Carlos Brown (General Surgery)
- Robert Cowan (OB/Gyn)
- Tamarah Duperval-Brownlee (Family Medicine)
- Byron Elliott (Perinatologist)
- Leighton Ellis (Pediatrics)
- David Fleeger (Colorectal Surgery)
- Declan Fleming (Surgical Oncology)
- Nilda Garcia (Pediatric Surgery)
- Osvaldo Gigliotti (Cardiology)
- Jennifer Goss (OB/Gyn)
- Sarmistha Hauger (Pediatric Infectious Disease)
- Louis Kennedy Hine (Internal Medicine)
- Stacy Jones (Anesthesia)
- Kathy Kraft
- Russell Krienke (Family Medicine)
- Anthony Manuel (Anesthesia)
- James Marroquin (Internal Medicine)
- Manuel Martin (Family Medicine)
- Alejandro Moreno (Internal Medicine)
- Bhin Pham (Gastroenterology)
- Andrew Reifsnyder (Radiology)
- Sarah Smiley (Internal Medicine)
- Said Soubra (Pulmonary / Critical Care)
- Diane Tyler (UT-Austin Nurse Practitioner Programs)
- Walkes Desmar
- Kari Wolf (Psychiatry)
- David Wright (Family Medicine)
- Karen Wright (Pediatric Cardiology)

DRAFT CHARGES

Expectation is that you will attend meetings, engage in dialog, and provide feedback as the steering committee representative's present information to the group.

Provide timely and accurate updates from the Steering Committee and Working Groups to the Austin Community, the Healthcare Community, and other key stakeholders

Gather input from community and stakeholders in order to facilitate transfer of information to the Dell Medical School leadership team and working groups

Provide consultation to the steering committee on curriculum development, interprofessional education initiatives, faculty development and other areas as needed.

COMMUNITY INVOLVEMENT TEAM

DRAFT MEMBERSHIP

- Greg Hartman **Co-Chair** (President/CEO, Seton UMCB)
- Amy Thomas **Co-Chair** (Vice Chancellor and Counsel for Health Affairs, UT System)
- W. Gaines Bagby (President, Rotary Club of Austin)
- Bathrop
- Terri Broussard Williams (Vice President of Government Relations, American Heart Association)
- Natalie Cofield (President/CEO, Capital City African American Chamber of Commerce)
- Gerald Davis (President/CEO, Goodwill)
- Gary Farmer (Chairman, Greater Austin Economic Development Corporation)
- Lynn Fowler (Executive Director, The Cain Foundation)
- Garbe
- Sandy Guzman (Legislative Director, Texas State Senator Kirk Watson)
- Greg Kozmetsky (Chairman, President & Treasurer, RGK Foundation)
- Kevin Lalande (Managing Director, Sante Ventures)
- Andy Martinez (President/CEO, Greater Austin Hispanic Chamber of Commerce)
- Earl Maxwell (St. David's Foundation)
- Rosie Mendoza (Board Chair, Central Health)
- Tom Meredith (Co-Founder, Waller Creek Conservancy)
- Janet Mountain (Executive Director, Michael & Susan Dell Foundation)
- David Pena, Jr. (President, Greater Austin Asian Chamber of Commerce)

- Melanie Plummer (Executive Director, Austin Young Chamber of Commerce)
- Dan Pruett (President/CEO, Meals on Wheels)
- Mike Rollins (President, Austin Chamber of Commerce)
- Martha Smiley (Counsel to the Firm Enoch Kever, PLLC)
- Tom Spencer (CEO, Interfaith Action of Central Texas)
- Leslie Sweet (Director of Public Affairs for Central Texas, HEB)
- Tim Taylor (Partner, Jackson Walker LLP, Austin Office)
- Doug Ulman (Chief Executive Officer, Livestrong Foundation)
- *Matt Winkler (Board Chairman, Asuragen)—Consult Only*

DRAFT CHARGES

Expectation is that you will attend meetings, engage in dialog, and provide feedback as the steering committee representative's present information to the group.

Provide timely and accurate updates from the Steering Committee and Working Groups to the Austin Community, the Healthcare Community, and other key stakeholders

Gather input from community and stakeholders in order to facilitate transfer of information to the Dell Medical School leadership team and working groups

Provide consultation to the steering committee on curriculum development, interprofessional education initiatives, faculty development and other areas as needed.

WOMAN'S HEALTH ENGAGEMENT GROUP:

DRAFT RECOMMENDATIONS FOR MEMBERSHIP CONSIDERATION

- Sue Cox—**Chair** (UTSW Regional Dean, Austin Programs)
- Amy Shaw Thomas (Vice Chancellor for Health Affairs, UT System)
- Sandy Guzman (Legislative Director, Texas State Senator Kirk Watson)
- Trish Young Brown (CEO Central Health)
- John Gianopoulos (President/CEO Seton Perinatal Services, Seton)
- Susan Heinzelman (Director, Center for Women's and Gender Studies, College of Liberal Arts)
- Judy Langlois (Vice Provost and Dean, Office of Graduate Studies, Department of Psychology, College of Liberal Arts)
- Janet Ellzey (Vice Provost, Dept Mechanical Engineering)
- Robin Ausley
- Two Local MDs (TBD)

DRAFT CHARGES

Expectation is that you will attend meetings, engage in dialog, and provide feedback as the steering committee representative's present information to the group.

Provide timely and accurate updates from the Steering Committee and Working Groups to the Austin Community, the Healthcare Community, and other key stakeholders

Gather input from community and stakeholders in order to facilitate transfer of information to the Dell Medical School leadership team and working groups

Provide consultation to the steering committee on curriculum development, interprofessional education initiatives, faculty development and other areas as needed.

INTERIM DEAN'S OFFICE:
ACADEMIC / CLINICAL AFFAIRS

STUDENT AFFAIRS / ADMISSIONS
- J. Scott Wright, PhD (Executive Director, Texas Medical and Dental School Application Process)
- Reg Baptiste (Assoc Dean, College of Natural Sciences)
- Lesley Riley (Program Director, College of Natural Sciences, UT Austin)

CURRICULUM—SUE COX

RESEARCH—BOB MESSING

FINANCIAL AFFAIRS:
- Kevin Hegarty (Vice President and Chief Financial Officer, UT Austin)
- Dan Slesnick (Senior Vice Provost for Resource Management, UT Austin)
- John Roan (Consultant)

ACCREDITATION: Point people
1. THECB—Mike Kerker (Associate Vice Provost, UT Austin)
2. LCME—Sue Cox (UTSW Regional Dean, Austin Programs)
3. James E Griffin—(consultant)
4. SACS—Neal Armstrong (Vice Provost, UT Austin)

COMMUNICATIONS:
- Gary Susswein (Director of University Media Relations, UT Austin)
- Tara Doolittle (Director of Media Outreach, UT Austin)

- Robert Cullick (Media Outreach, UT Austin)
- Christie Garbe (Vice President of Planning & Communications, Central Health)
- Adrienne Lallo (Seton Communications Director)
- Randa Safady (Vice Chancellor for External Relations, UT System) or designee

Dell Medical School at UT Austin Mission, Vision, Core Values, and Goals, March 27, 2013

Dell Medical School at UT Austin
Mission, Vision, Core Values, and Goals
March 2013

Mission:

The University of Texas at Austin Dell Medical School is committed to improving human health through excellence in interprofessional and trans-disciplinary education, research, healthcare and community involvement.

Vision:

The School will:

- Transform current and future medicine and the healthcare delivery system through discovery, innovation, application, and translation.

- Educate and inspire the next generation of physician leaders by providing the foundation for our students to become skillful, ethical, and compassionate physicians; inquisitive scientists who are committed to the scholarship of discovery; and dynamic and successful medical educators.

- Prepare clinicians to provide person-centered, high-quality, safe and cost-effective care that leads to optimal outcomes for the communities we serve.

- Advance boundaries of medicine by being a vanguard of research and by creating an environment of scholarship, intellectual curiosity and exchange.

- Foster interprofessional team development to enhance patient safety and improve healthcare outcomes.

Core Values:

The school will accomplish its Mission and Vision by modeling

- Adaptability – maintain flexibility and resilience in order to respond to changing needs and expectations of individuals and the community

- Collaboration – work together and align interprofessional teams to fulfill our mission regardless of organizational boundaries

- Compassion - relate to others in a caring, empathic manner and strive to prevent and relieve suffering.

1

- Discovery – motivate towards the cutting edge of what is unknown by empowering our faculty and students to remain intellectually curious and inquisitive

- Diversity –create, foster, and maintain a culturally diverse learning community

- Excellence - achieve our highest goals and become the best we can be

- Integrity – maintain the highest respect, trust and ethical standards in all our interactions and activities

- Leadership – educate and train physicians, researchers, and other healthcare professionals to become leaders in their fields at a regional, state and national level

- Learning – develop strategies for life-long, self-directed learning, sharing of knowledge, and translating new concepts to practice

- Responsibility - exhibit a strong sense of duty, stewardship and accountability to each other and to our varied constituencies.

Priority Goals:

- Achieve accreditation with state and national licensing bodies to admit the first class of 50 medical students by mid-2016

- Create a curriculum using modern technologies and teaching methods that foster self-directed, intellectually curious, and lifelong learning

- Leverage the strong science, engineering, social science, and professional degree programs at UT Austin to provide medical students, residents, and fellows opportunities to pursue trans-disciplinary research and joint/ dual degrees.

2

UT Austin Medical School Summary Sources and Uses of Funds, Preliminary

U.T. Austin Medical School, Summary Sources and Uses of Funds

($ millions)	FY13	FY14	FY15	FY16	FY17
Estimated Sources of Funds					
Practice Plan	—	24.5	35.2	52.2	70.5
State Formula Funding	—	—	0.8	1.0	1.0
Other Seton Contribution	21.8	88.3	114.9	122.2	124.7
Subtotal-Clinical	21.8	112.8	150.9	175.4	196.2
Hospital District	35.0	35.0	35.0	35.0	35.0
Grants		6.9	12.8	19.5	28.8
State Formula Funding		—	—	—	2.5
State Resident Supervision		—	—	—	0.7
Seton		10.4	18.4	34.0	36.4
Tuition and Fees		—	—	—	0.8
Philanthropy		—	—	—	—
Regents STARS Funding (PUF)	5.0	5.0	5.0	5.0	5.0
Regents Funding (AUF)	25.0	25.0	25.0	25.0	25.0
Subtotal-Non Clinical	65.0	82.3	96.1	118.6	134.2
Total Estimated Sources	86.80	195.05	247.04	293.95	330.40
Estimated Uses of Funds					
Resident Program	21.8	24.2	26.9	30.2	35.1
Clinical Program	—	88.6	124.0	145.2	161.1
Subtotal Clinical	21.8	112.8	150.9	175.4	196.2
Non-clinical Operations	1.2	52.2	81.7	119.9	143.5
Total Estimated Uses	23.0	165.0	232.6	295.2	339.7
Operations Positive/(Negative)	63.8	30.1	14.4	(1.3)	(9.3)
Cumulative Operations	63.8	93.9	108.3	107.0	97.8

Note: Preliminary—For Discussion Purposes Only

FY18	FY19	FY20	FY21	FY22	FY23	FY24	Total	Average
84.1	93.1	99.6	105.1	111.1	117.6	124.1	917.1	76.4
1.1	1.1	1.4	1.4	1.6	1.6	1.7	12.8	1.1
124.4	128.2	137.5	149.5	161.2	171.3	179.7	1,523.7	127.0
209.6	222.4	238.5	256.0	273.9	290.5	305.6	2,453.5	204.5
35.0	35.0	35.0	35.0	35.0	35.0	35.0	420.0	35.0
32.5	37.6	41.6	54.0	69.1	77.7	89.0	469.6	42.7
2.6	2.6	8.0	8.0	14.1	14.1	15.0	66.9	6.1
0.9	0.9	1.0	1.0	1.3	1.3	1.4	8.5	0.8
34.7	29.9	32.2	34.7	37.1	39.5	41.5	348.6	31.7
1.1	1.1	2.2	3.5	4.8	6.3	6.9	26.7	2.4
—	—	—	—	—	—	—	—	—
5.0	2.5	—	—	—	—	—	32.5	2.7
25.0	25.0	25.0	25.0	25.0	25.0	25.0	300.0	25.0
136.8	134.5	145.0	161.2	186.4	198.8	213.9	1,672.8	139.4
346.41	356.90	383.54	417.19	460.26	489.32	519.42	4,126.3	343.9
41.1	46.7	52.3	57.9	63.5	68.0	71.8	539.5	45.0
168.6	175.7	186.2	198.1	210.3	222.5	233.7	1,914.0	159.5
209.6	222.4	238.5	256.0	273.9	290.5	305.6	2,453.5	204.5
162.4	171.0	163.8	169.5	180.8	190.7	204.3	1,641.01	136.7
372.0	393.4	402.3	425.5	454.7	481.2	509.9	4,094.4	341.2
(25.6)	(36.5)	(18.8)	(8.3)	5.6	8.1	9.6	31.9	2.7
72.1	35.6	16.8	8.6	14.2	22.3	31.9		

APPENDIX 18

Institution or Medical School?
A Comparison of the Options

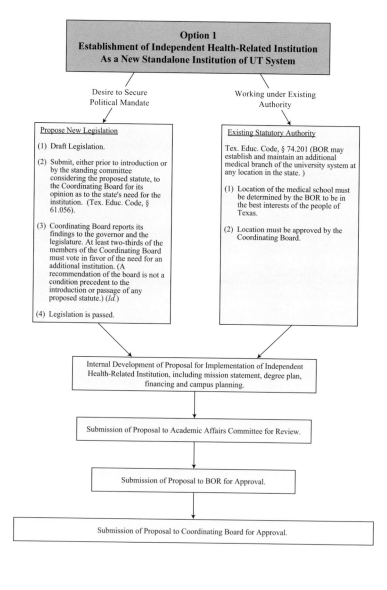

Option 1
Establishment of Independent Health-Related Institution
As a New Standalone Institution of UT System

Desire to Secure
Political Mandate

Working under Existing
Authority

Propose New Legislation

(1) Draft Legislation.

(2) Submit, either prior to introduction or
by the standing committee
considering the proposed statute, to
the Coordinating Board for its
opinion as to the state's need for the
institution. (Tex. Educ. Code, §
61.056).

(3) Coordinating Board reports its
findings to the governor and the
legislature. At least two-thirds of the
members of the Coordinating Board
must vote in favor of the need for an
additional institution. (A
recommendation of the board is not a
condition precedent to the
introduction or passage of any
proposed statute.) (*Id.*)

(4) Legislation is passed.

Existing Statutory Authority

Tex. Educ. Code, § 74.201 (BOR may
establish and maintain an additional
medical branch of the university system at
any location in the state.)

(1) Location of the medical school must
be determined by the BOR to be in
the best interests of the people of
Texas.

(2) Location must be approved by the
Coordinating Board.

Internal Development of Proposal for Implementation of Independent
Health-Related Institution, including mission statement, degree plan,
financing and campus planning.

Submission of Proposal to Academic Affairs Committee for Review.

Submission of Proposal to BOR for Approval.

Submission of Proposal to Coordinating Board for Approval.

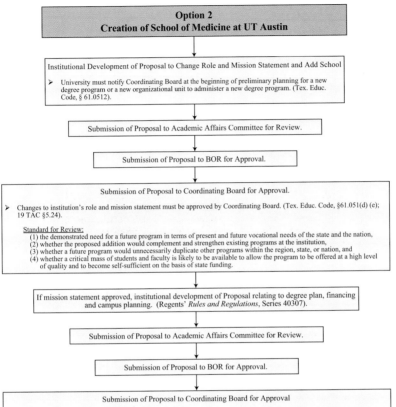

Option 2
Creation of School of Medicine at UT Austin

Institutional Development of Proposal to Change Role and Mission Statement and Add School

➢ University must notify Coordinating Board at the beginning of preliminary planning for a new degree program or a new organizational unit to administer a new degree program. (Tex. Educ. Code, § 61.0512).

Submission of Proposal to Academic Affairs Committee for Review.

Submission of Proposal to BOR for Approval.

Submission of Proposal to Coordinating Board for Approval.

➢ Changes to institution's role and mission statement must be approved by Coordinating Board. (Tex. Educ. Code, §61.051(d) (e); 19 TAC §5.24).

Standard for Review:
(1) the demonstrated need for a future program in terms of present and future vocational needs of the state and the nation,
(2) whether the proposed addition would complement and strengthen existing programs at the institution,
(3) whether a future program would unnecessarily duplicate other programs within the region, state, or nation, and
(4) whether a critical mass of students and faculty is likely to be available to allow the program to be offered at a high level of quality and to become self-sufficient on the basis of state funding.

If mission statement approved, institutional development of Proposal relating to degree plan, financing and campus planning. (Regents' *Rules and Regulations*, Series 40307).

Submission of Proposal to Academic Affairs Committee for Review.

Submission of Proposal to BOR for Approval.

Submission of Proposal to Coordinating Board for Approval

➢ No new department, school, degree program, or certificate program may be added at any public institution of higher education except with specific prior approval of the Coordinating Board. (Tex. Educ. Code, §§61.051(e) and 65.31(b); 19 TAC §5.46).

Criteria for Approval of New Doctoral Programs: Includes design of the program, need for the program, freedom of inquiry and expression, faculty resources, critical mass of superior students, on-campus residency expectations, adequate financial assistance for doctoral students, carefully planned program of study, program evaluation standards, and library resources.

➢ Financing. A new department, school, or degree or certificate program may not be initiated by any institution of higher education until the Coordinating Board has made a written finding that the department, school, or degree or certificate program is adequately financed. (Tex. Educ. Code, §§ 61.054 and 61.055; 19 TAC §5.49).

➢ Campus Planning. Coordinating Board must approve all new construction of buildings and facilities at institutions. (Tex. Educ. Code, §§61.0572, 61.058, and §61.0582; 19 TAC §17.1, et. seq).

➢ Unless otherwise stipulated at the time of approval, a new degree program approved by the Coordinating Board must be established within two years of approval, otherwise its approval is no longer valid. (19 TAC 5.4(b)).

"Watson Emphasizing Goal, Not Cost, When It Comes to Medical School," by Ralph K. M. Haurwitz and Mary Ann Roser, *Austin American-Statesman*, September 20, 2011

WATSON EMPHASIZING GOAL, NOT COST, WHEN IT COMES TO MEDICAL SCHOOL

By Ralph K.M. Haurwitz and Mary Ann Roser

American-Statesman Staff

Statesman.com

Tuesday, Sept. 20, 2011

The 10-year, 10-point to-do list offered by state Sen. Kirk Watson to advance medical education, research and treatment in Austin is fairly straightforward:

Establish a medical school at the University of Texas. Build a new teaching hospital. Open a comprehensive cancer treatment center. Expand mental health services. Modernize community health clinics. Bolster the Travis County medical examiner's office. And so on.

Just don't ask how much it all might cost. That, the Democrat from Austin said repeatedly, is premature.

"We have yet to map out what will be a complex path so that we'll be able to make the sort of investment decisions, philanthropic decisions, whatever economic decisions need to be made," Watson said. "And I refuse to allow this program to—and I'll say it again—literally jump to conclusions until we have mapped out that complex path."

Watson outlined his plan Tuesday at a luncheon organized by the Real Estate Council of Austin at the Four Seasons Hotel. Achieving the goals, he said, would be on a par with Austin's emergence as a high-tech hub. And if Austin fails to act, it will miss out on enormous benefits to the region's health care, economy and quality of life, he said.

The civic, education, business and political figures in the audience gave the senator a standing ovation. Gov. Rick Perry, a Republican, also supports the concept of a medical school, according to his spokeswoman.

"If we can achieve this, it will be the biggest thing to happen in the City of Austin in my lifetime," said Mayor Lee Leffingwell, named by Watson to an organizing committee charged with mapping out the details. Watson will serve as the panel's chairman.

A medical school, which has been under discussion for years, is the committee's first goal. "We're going to get this done," said panel member Francisco Cigarroa, chancellor of the University of Texas System, who has made expansion of medical education in Austin and South Texas top priorities.

Like Watson, Cigarroa declined to be drawn into a detailed discussion about what it might cost to develop a medical school here. However, Kenneth Shine, the system's executive vice chancellor for health affairs, said that his estimate of $1 billion to $2 billion seven years ago is no longer operative.

Substantial investment has already been made by the Seton Healthcare Family, which has shouldered faculty and other costs in recent years for medical training here in conjunction with the Dallas-based UT Southwestern Medical Center, he said.

Seton officials began earlier this year to speak publicly of a goal of replacing the aging University Medical Center Brackenridge, the community's safety-net hospital and home of the region's trauma center.

Watson's pairing of a medical school with a state-of-the-art teaching hospital puts those plans on a 10-year timetable, said Greg Hartman, president and CEO of UMC Brackenridge and Seton Medical Center Austin. "It puts the fuel in the tank to make it happen," he said.

Seton operates the publicly owned hospital near the UT campus for Central Health, Travis County's health care district. Hartman said he expected that Seton would play "a significant role," along with Central Health, in financing a replacement hospital.

Central Health is in general agreement that a new hospital is needed, said Patricia Young Brown, its president and CEO. "We've talked about that from the beginning" of the hospital district's formation by voters in 2004, she said.

Clarke Heidrick, a Central Health board member since the hospital district's inception, said he and other board members are excited about working with Watson to establish a medical school and to determine Central Health's role in that effort. "I hope we'll contribute financially if that makes sense," Heidrick said.

Central Health has a $42 million reserve account that can be used for one-time or ongoing expenditures to correct budget deficits.

STATE SEN. KIRK WATSON'S 10 GOALS

1. Build a medical school in Austin with everything from student housing to faculty members who would teach and also treat patients.
2. Build a modern teaching hospital to replace University Medical Center Brackenridge.
3. Modernize community health clinics whose patients would include those lacking health insurance.
4. Develop a research institute by building on the collaboration between the Seton Healthcare Family and the University of Texas System.
5. Launch a technology incubator to commercialize scientific discoveries.
6. Start a comprehensive cancer treatment center.
7. Provide psychiatric care and facilities that include crisis centers, emergency care and services aimed at reducing adolescent suicide.
8. Improve water lines and other infrastructure in the area around Brackenridge, Waterloo Park and Waller Creek so an area near Interstate 35 may "be planned in a way that allows old barriers to be torn down, and communities that have been wrongly split ... to be connected."
9. Strengthen the medical examiner's office by allowing medical students and doctors to train there.
10. Resolve funding for a medical school, the No. 1. stumbling block to building one.

ORGANIZING COMMITTEE MEMBERS

University of Texas System Chancellor Francisco Cigarroa and Executive Vice Chancellor Kenneth Shine

UT Southwestern Medical Center Regional Dean for Austin Programs Sue Cox

UT-Austin President William Powers Jr. and Executive Vice President and Provost Steven Leslie

Seton Healthcare Family President and CEO Charles Barnett

St. David's HealthCare President and CEO David Huffstutler

Central Health Board Chairman Tom Coopwood and incoming Chairwoman Rosie Mendoza

Austin Community Foundation President and CEO Jeff Garvey

Greater Austin Chamber of Commerce Incoming Chairman Clarke Heidrick, also on the Central Health board

Travis County Medical Society representatives (to be named)

Health clinic representatives (to be named)

Livestrong Foundation CEO Doug Ulman

City of Austin Mayor Lee Leffingwell

Travis County Judge Sam Biscoe

Board of Regents Motion on Development of a Medical School, May 3, 2012

Presented to the Board
May 3, 2012

Vice Chairman Hicks

MOTION FROM OPEN SESSION
May 3, 2012

I move that the U. T. System Board of Regents

a.   commit to the development of a medical school in Austin;

b.   commit additional Available University Fund monies toward the creation of a medical school at U. T. Austin, equal to the greater of $25 million annually or a 3% increase in the annual AUF distribution to U. T. Austin from 45 to 48%; and

c.   approve the allocation of $5 million of STARS recruiting monies, per year, for eight years, to U. T. Austin as additional support to create the medical school at U. T. Austin.

I further move that the financial commitments of the Board of Regents be contingent upon the continuation of the Seton Healthcare Family support of graduate medical education residency programs and clinical faculty positions at current or increased levels and the availability of reliable and continuing funding of $35 million annually from local community sources for the direct support of a medical school at U. T. Austin.

I also move that the Board of Regents review the funding streams to support the medical school 10 years after its establishment consistent with the Board's fiduciary responsibilities.

Austin Medical School

Proposition 1, Central Health Tax Ratification Election, Travis County Central Health District, November 6, 2012

PROPOSITION 1

OFFICIAL BALLOT LANGUAGE:

Approving the ad valorem tax rate of $0.129 per $100 valuation in Central Health, also known as the Travis County Healthcare District, for the 2013 tax year, a rate that exceeds the district's rollback tax rate. The proposed ad valorem tax rate exceeds the ad valorem tax rate most recently adopted by the district by $0.05 per $100 valuation; funds will be used for improved healthcare in Travis County, including support for a new medical school consistent with the mission of Central Health, a site for a new teaching hospital, trauma services, specialty medicine such as cancer care, community-wide health clinics, training for physicians, nurses and other healthcare professionals, primary care, behavioral and mental healthcare, prevention and wellness programs, and/or to obtain federal matching funds for healthcare services.

Chancellor's Message on Establishing a Medical School at UT Austin, November 1, 2012

CHANCELLOR'S MESSAGE

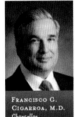

FRANCISCO G.
CIGARROA, M.D.
Chancellor

The University of Texas System is on the verge of a once-in-a-generation milestone – establishing a medical school at The University of Texas at Austin. Already, UT Austin is an undisputed Tier 1 research institution with a global reputation for excellence. Just a few weeks ago, UT Austin was ranked among the top 25 universities in the *Times Higher Education World University Rankings*.

A school of medicine at UT Austin will enhance the university's reputation and position it in an even stronger stance to compete for the very best faculty, graduate students, scientists, grants, philanthropy, technology commercialization opportunities and public/private partnerships.

The medical school at UT Austin would be the first, and only, comprehensive, research-intensive school of medicine on an academic campus in Texas. Such a move would complement many of UT Austin's programs, including natural sciences, nursing, social work, pharmacy and engineering. We have a unique opportunity right now to design a medical school that is a research- intensive institution combined with strong, community-based educational experiences.

While there is no doubt that UT Austin will benefit from a medical school on campus, it is Texans who will receive the ultimate advantage. There are significant physician shortages in Texas -- a situation we want to remedy by creating more medical school and residency slots. UT System leaders are working aggressively and successfully with private hospital partners to increase the number of residency positions, both around the state and in Austin. We know that if a medical student does his or her training in Texas and stays in state for their residency education, there is an 82 percent chance they will remain in Texas to practice medicine. Texas needs more doctors and we want to satisfy that need.

A medical school at UT Austin will also provide great benefits to the local community. Central Health plans to contract with the medical school for services and is designing an innovative, community-based model. Professionals will train for careers in medicine by delivering patient-based care throughout Travis County, creating a partnership that will focus on keeping people healthy across Central Texas.

Why is public support necessary? The UT System Board of Regents has committed to a significant financial investment – $25 million a year in perpetuity, and an additional $5 million a year for eight years to purchase equipment -- from the Permanent University Fund for a medical school at UT Austin. PUF funds have to support many initiatives at 15 UT institutions, including those that keep UT Austin ranked among the best universities in the world. Additional support is necessary to pay for health services and improve quality and access to healthcare throughout Central Texas.

Texas has a rich history of public support and partnership to bring medical schools to cities that need them. Health institutions around the state receive a range of support from hospital districts in Dallas, Houston and San Antonio. Many medical centers, schools and research facilities were founded on land donated by cities or foundations. More than 50 years ago, a combination of county bonds, free land and other incentives were used to bring a medical school to San Antonio. Voters in El Paso passed a $120 million bond issue in 2007 to build a children's hospital and the El Paso City Council earmarks about $3.2 million annually from fees paid by electric utility customers for healthcare and economic development.

This is yet another historic moment for the University of Texas at Austin. A medical school will catapult the university to rank among the most elite schools in the country and the world, while at the same time meeting essential healthcare needs for Austin residents and growing a much-needed population of doctors to care for Texans across the state.

With great respect,

Francisco G. Cigarroa, M.D.

"UT Medical School Should Be 'World-Class,' Powers Says," by Ralph K. M. Haurwitz, *Austin American-Statesman*, October 6, 2011

UT MEDICAL SCHOOL SHOULD BE 'WORLD-CLASS,' POWERS SAYS

By Ralph K.M. Haurwitz
Posted Oct 7, 2011 at 12:01 AM

The University of Texas wants to establish a "world-class medical school," the university's president said Thursday.

"It will add to the health care of the city," said UT President William Powers Jr. "It will spark the biotech arena. The benefits are absolutely tremendous."

He spoke at a gathering hosted by Leadership Austin, a nonprofit civic organization, at the Long Center for the Performing Arts. Joining him on the stage in extolling the economic and health benefits of a medical school were state Sen. Kirk Watson, D-Austin, and Jesus Garza, executive vice president and chief operating officer of the Seton Healthcare Family.

Powers said the medical school should be on the quality level of such top schools as the UT Southwestern Medical Center in Dallas and UCLA's medical school.

He said a number of important elements are already in place at the Austin flagship, including programs in biomedical engineering, chemistry, nursing, pharmacy and social work. Likening a medical school to an iceberg, Powers described those elements as "the big part of the iceberg."

He declined to estimate how much a building for educating medical students might cost.

The UT president first endorsed the notion of a medical school during his state of the university address last month. About two weeks earlier, the UT System

Board of Regents approved Chancellor Francisco Cigarroa's goal along the same lines, for four-year "research intensive medical education, including expanded residencies, biomedical research and interdisciplinary health education in Austin."

Watson, a former Austin mayor, has established an organizing committee to work toward establishing a medical school. Powers is a member of the panel, which also includes representatives from Seton, the UT System, St. David's HealthCare, local governments and philanthropic groups.

Memorandum of Understanding, UT Austin, Central Health, Seton, and the Community Care Collaborative, July 25, 2013

**MEMORANDUM OF UNDERSTANDING BETWEEN
THE UNIVERSITY OF TEXAS AT AUSTIN, CENTRAL HEALTH, SETON,
AND THE COMMUNITY CARE COLLABORATIVE**

This is a Memorandum of Understanding ("MOU") between Travis County Healthcare District d/b/a Central Health, ("Central Health"), The University of Texas at Austin ("UT"), the Community Care Collaborative ("CCC"), and Seton Family of Hospitals ("Seton") regarding their mutual desire and intention to collaborate to transform and improve health care for all residents in Travis County including those who are uninsured by, among other things, creating an integrated delivery system (the "IDS"), expanding the medical services available in Travis County, and increasing the number and quality of physicians in Travis County. The parties enter into this MOU with the understanding that the foundations for transformative improvement in health care include the establishment of a medical school at UT (the "Medical School"). UT has agreed to build and operate the Medical School in Austin in reliance on a stable recurring commitment of $35 million annually, consistent with the Travis County voters' November 2012 approval of Proposition I. Consequently, because it is in the best interests of the various populations they serve, the parties are entering into this MOU with the intention of entering into more formal arrangements. Central Health, the CCC, Seton, and UT are individually referred to as "party" and collectively referred to as "parties." The effective date of this MOU is August 30, 2013 ("Effective Date").

      1.   Improving Care in Travis County. The parties have agreed to collaborate and pool their resources to improve the health care delivery system in Travis County. The parties' intentions are as follows:

      a.   Seton will build and operate a new teaching hospital that will be part of Seton's and Central Health's indigent and charity care safety net system;

      b.   Seton and Central Health, individually and through the CCC, will expand and add new medical services in Travis County to serve the indigent and medical access program ("MAP") populations;

      c.   UT will build and operate the Medical School in Travis County with a focus on patient centered interprofessional education and health care and leading edge basic and translational research to advance the quality of health care;

      d.   Seton will affiliate with UT's Medical School to support faculty and to train students and residents at the teaching hospital that will improve and expand the medical care services in Travis County available to indigent and MAP populations; and

      e.   Central Health and the CCC will incorporate the Medical School's faculty, students, and residents into the IDS.

      2.   Central Health's and Seton's Support for the IDS and the Medical School.

a.   UT acknowledges that in order to achieve the goal of bettering indigent and MAP care in Travis County, Seton and Central Health have entered into a "Master Agreement" effective June 1, 2013.

b.   UT acknowledges that Central Health, Seton, and the CCC are expecting that UT will develop and establish a new Medical School at the Austin campus of UT. UT has taken the initial steps to establish this new Medical School and intends to move forward with this initiative with the expectation of enrolling an initial class of students in 2016.

c.   UT further acknowledges that a critical element to the new IDS is the decision by Seton and Central Health to jointly form and fund a Texas non-profit corporation, the CCC, consistent with the Master Agreement. The parties intend for the CCC to be the main vehicle through which they will invest in new medical resources and services in Travis County for the indigent and MAP populations and to transition into an IDS.

d.   The parties acknowledge and agree that there are certain investments ("Permitted Investments") that would both support the IDS and benefit UT and would comply with all legal and regulatory restrictions applicable to the party making the investment and the party receiving the benefit of the investment. It is acknowledged and agreed that such investments are intended for the purpose of providing operating support of the Medical School that will facilitate and enhance the recruitment and work of its faculty, researchers, administrators, and clinicians. "Permitted Investments" are needed and intended to augment clinical services for Travis County residents, benefit overall health care by educating and training future physicians, discover new knowledge that enhances health and health care, make available medical innovations to the Travis County population, and provide collaborative and integrated medical care.

e.   For UT fiscal years beginning on or after the Effective Date, CCC will, as its first annual priority, cause $35 million to be paid to UT each fiscal year to be used by UT for one or more Permitted Investments as determined in the sole and exclusive discretion of UT ("Permitted Investment Payment"). To the extent permitted by the Constitution and laws of the State of Texas, Central Health will guarantee such annual payments to be made to UT by CCC or otherwise.

3.   No Violation of Law & Enforceability. The parties all agree that nothing in this MOU or any agreement arising out of this MOU will obligate the parties to take any action that would violate the laws of the State of Texas or the United States. The parties agree that this MOU is only the expression of intent by the parties and, except as otherwise provided herein, is not enforceable until the definitive documents are created.

4.   Approvals. This MOU is not legally enforceable and is not a binding obligation or agreement between the parties. The parties acknowledge and agree that they cannot and will

DMSLIBRARY01:21257136.1

not reach any legally enforceable and binding agreement until each of their respective governing boards has approved such agreement, if necessary, and such agreement has been properly executed. In addition, this MOU does not create any legally enforceable or binding obligation on any party to execute any final enforceable agreements.

5.   Expenses. Each party will pay its own expenses and costs incidental to the negotiation and completion of the documents intended to formalize and implement the understandings set forth in this MOU.

6.   Effective Date. This MOU will remain in effect from the Effective Date through the execution by the parties of the enforceable and binding agreement referred to in Section 4. Any party may terminate this MOU at any time in its own discretion by written notice to the other parties.

7.   Counterparts. This MOU may be executed in counterparts, each of which shall be original but which together shall constitute one and the same instrument.

IN WITNESS WHEREOF, the parties hereto have caused this MOU to be executed by their duly authorized officers, all as of the dates written below.

THE UNIVERSITY OF TEXAS AT AUSTIN

By:
Name: WILLIAM POWERS
Title: PRESIDENT

Date: 9/26/13

SETON FAMILY OF HOSPITALS

By:
Name: Jesús Garza
Title: President and Chief Executive Officer – Seton Healthcare Family

Date: 9-24-2013

TRAVIS COUNTY HEALTHCARE DISTRICT
D/B/A CENTRAL HEALTH

By:
Name: Rosie Mendoza
Title: Chairperson of the Board

Date: 08/27/2013

COMMUNITY CARE COLLABORATIVE

By:
Name:
Title: ED

Date: 9/6/2013

Press Release on Organization and Governance and Medical School Dean Search, April 11, 2013

PRESS RELEASE

Thursday, April 11, 2013

COMMITTEE LAUNCHES SEARCH FOR DELL MEDICAL SCHOOL FOUNDING DEAN

AUSTIN, Texas—A committee of 18 educators, community leaders, health professionals and students has begun the search for a founding dean of the Dell Medical School, the first new medical school among top-ranked research universities in more than 35 years.

"This is a tremendous opportunity for the university, the community and most of all, for a very talented person who will serve as inaugural dean to build the Dell Medical School from the ground up," said Steven Leslie, executive vice president and provost for The University of Texas at Austin.

"In Austin, we have a unique situation," Leslie said. "Major public and private institutions are coming together and will construct the laboratories and classrooms of a medical school along with a new teaching hospital. At the same time, community programs will be initiated to serve people who need health care. There will be tremendous interest from dean candidates who want to make a difference in the health of a community and an impact on global health concerns."

Dean search committees typically comprise deans, professors and students. The Dell Medical School founding dean search committee includes these and also has members from key organizations such as Seton Healthcare Family and Central Health, partners in the initiative, as well as a community physician.

Seton is constructing a new teaching hospital; Central Health has been authorized by the public to purchase services for uninsured Travis County residents from the hospital. Two medical schools UT Health Science Center at San Antonio and UT Southwestern Medical School also are represented.

The university has engaged Witt/Kieffer, a search firm with extensive experience identifying deans for medical and health sciences schools including nursing, dentistry, allied health, pharmacy, veterinary medicine, public health and biomedical/life sciences.

Chairing the committee will be Dr. Robert O. Messing, vice provost for biomedical sciences and the Henry M. Burlage Centennial Endowed Professor in Pharmacy. Messing came to the university in January from the University of California, San Francisco, where he was on the faculty for 26 years, having spent the past 15 years as an administrator helping to build a highly successful research institute, the Ernest Gallo Clinic and Research Center.

"The founding dean will be someone who can create a medical program that graduates doctors who are intellectually curious and inspired by their years studying with professors in many diverse disciplines," Messing said. "During their careers, these doctors will make a difference in how medicine is practiced and taught."

The committee hopes to have a dean in place in time for the start of the new academic year in order to prepare for the first class of about 50 students, who are expected to matriculate in 2016.

The members of the search committee are:

MEMBER	AFFILIATION
Robert O. Messing, Chair	Vice Provost for Biomedical Sciences
Reginald C. Baptiste	Capital Cardiothoracic Surgeons
Da'marcus E. Baymon	Senior, UT Austin College of Natural Sciences
Susan Cox	UT Southwestern Regional Dean for Austin Programs
Lynn Crismon	Dean, UT Austin College of Pharmacy
Greg Fenves	Dean, UT Austin Cockrell School of Engineering
J. Gregory Fitz	Executive Vice President for Academic Affairs and Provost, Dean of UT Southwestern Medical School
Jesús Garza	President and Chief Executive Officer, Seton Healthcare Family
Francisco González-Scarano	Dean of the School of Medicine and Vice President for Medical Affairs at the UT Health Science Center at San Antonio
Andrea Gore	Professor, College of Pharmacy

Clarke Heidrick	Central Health Board of Managers
Linda Hicke	Dean, UT Austin College of Natural Sciences
Dan Johnston	Chair of Neurobiology Section, UT Austin College of Natural Sciences
Alan Lambowitz	Director of the Institute for Cellular and Molecular Biology, UT Austin
James O. Lindsey	Senior Vice President, Medical Affairs and Chief Medical Officer, Seton Healthcare Family
Russell Poldrack	Director, Imaging Research Center, UT Austin College of Liberal Arts
Stephanie Tutak	Junior, UT Austin College of Natural Sciences
Mary Velasquez	Associate Dean for Research, UT Austin School of Social Work

Inaugural Dean Position Specification, June 2013

THE UNIVERSITY OF

TEXAS

AT AUSTIN

Inaugural Dean - Dell Medical School
Position Specification

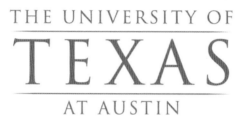

Teaching, Healing, Advancing Health.

WITT / KIEFFER
Leaders Connecting Leaders

Prepared by

John K. Thornburgh
Brian C. Bloomfield
Michael M.E. Johns, M.D.

June, 2013

The Opportunity

The Dell Medical School of The University of Texas at Austin ("Dell Medical School") is seeking an exceptional leader to serve as its Inaugural Dean and quickly build this new enterprise into a world-renowned center for teaching, research, and clinical care.

Scheduled to accept its first class of 50 students in 2016, the new school intends to offer a unique opportunity in medical education. As part of the campus of one of the nation's leading research universities, it will pursue excellence in healthcare research and in transdisciplinary and interprofessional education. The Dell Medical School will be the fifth medical school in the UT System and the first medical school established in nearly five decades by a member of the Association of American Universities, an organization of leading public and private research universities.

As part of a visionary partnership with Seton Healthcare Family, a regional health care system, and Central Health, a public health care district, a new teaching hospital will be constructed adjacent to the new Dell Medical School. By designing these facilities concurrently within an integrated complex, the effort represents an unprecedented opportunity to create the best possible environment to respond to community needs and provide patient care.

An extraordinary commitment of resources has already been made to enable the development and success of the Dell Medical School. Seton Healthcare expects to invest $250 million towards the establishment of the teaching hospital. Central Health will leverage a recent publicly approved real estate levy with federal matching funds to provide $35 million in annual revenues to the project. The University of Texas System Board of Regents has pledged at least $25 million annually plus an additional $5 million per year for eight years, for faculty recruitment and support. Finally, the Michael & Susan Dell Foundation recently announced a $50 million gift to the school.

The Inaugural Dean will build collaborative relationships and innovative programs; recruit an outstanding faculty and staff; organize and direct the process leading to accreditation of the new school; oversee the completion of the new medical school facilities; and expand and build upon the partnerships in this uniquely pivotal venture. This Dean will have an unparalleled opportunity to lead the programmatic and physical construction of a new medical school that deploys state-of-the art facilities for basic and translational research, advanced technologies and the most advanced teaching and learning methods for a contemporary curriculum. The Dean will provide vision and leadership in advanced patient treatment and novel medical technologies. The Dean will show understanding of the global needs in health care. In addition, the Dean will have a unique opportunity to establish a strong entrepreneurial and innovation-culture in one of the most economically dynamic regions of the country.

The successful Inaugural Dean candidate will possess a medical degree from an accredited medical school and a substantial record of leadership and achievement in academic medicine, medical education, and medical research. The Dean must demonstrate the ability to effectively steward medical school resources; understand, appreciate and wisely guide the development of the medical education and research programs; effectively support the distinct academic and clinical partnerships; be able to represent the medical school in the various regional and national communities; and successfully raise funds from a variety of sources including private philanthropy.

Because the role of the Dean is new, complex and demanding, the successful candidate's experience must include progressively more responsible administrative experience in environments that rely upon vision, teamwork, planning, delegation of authority and measures of accountability. Above all, the Dean should present a scientific vision, and an entrepreneurial style and a track record of success in establishing new enterprises and leading through times of change.

This role presents the right leader with the opportunity to forge an historic cooperation among teachers, researchers and health care providers in state-of-the-art facilities, in a common effort to produce the knowledge, management systems and skilled doctors who will improve the lives of millions of people, both locally and globally.

The University of Texas at Austin

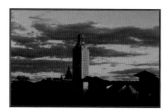

The University of Texas at Austin is one of the largest public universities in the United States and is the largest institution of The University of Texas System.

Founded in 1883, the university has grown from a single building, eight teachers, two departments and 221 students to a 350-acre main campus with 17 colleges and schools, about 24,000 faculty and staff, and more than 50,000 students.

The university's reach goes far beyond the borders of the main campus with satellite campuses and research centers across Texas, including the J.J. Pickle Research Campus, the Marine Science Institute, the McDonald Observatory, the Montopolis Research Center and the Brackenridge tract.

With an enrollment of 11,000 students and more than 3,500 master's and doctor's degrees awarded annually, the Graduate School is a national leader in graduate degrees awarded and one of the largest graduate schools in the nation. More than 8,700 bachelor's degrees are awarded annually in more than 170 fields of study and 100 majors.

The university has one of the most diverse student populations in the country and is a national leader in the number of undergraduate degrees awarded to minority students.

The Dell Medical School: An Overview

Mission, Vision and Values

Mission

The University of Texas at Austin Dell Medical School is committed to improving human health through excellence in interprofessional and transdisciplinary education, research, health care, and community involvement.

Vision

The School will:

- Transform current and future medicine and the health care delivery system through discovery, innovation, application, and translation.
- Educate and inspire the next generation of physician leaders by providing the foundation for our students to become skillful, ethical, and compassionate physicians; inquisitive scientists who are committed to the scholarship of discovery; and dynamic and successful medical educators.
- Prepare clinicians to provide person-centered, high-quality, safe and cost-effective care that leads to optimal outcomes for the communities we serve.
- Advance boundaries of medicine by being a vanguard of research and by creating an environment of scholarship, intellectual curiosity and exchange.
- Foster interprofessional team development to enhance patient safety and improve health care outcomes.
- Leverage clinical and research capabilities through collaboration with community healthcare providers and biotech businesses.

Core Values

The school will accomplish its Mission and Vision by modeling:

- Adaptability – maintain flexibility and resilience in order to respond to changing needs and expectations of individuals and the community.
- Collaboration – work together and align interprofessional teams to fulfill our mission regardless of organizational boundaries.
- Compassion - relate to others in a caring, empathic manner and strive to prevent and relieve suffering.
- Discovery – motivate towards the cutting edge of what is unknown by empowering our faculty and students to remain intellectually curious and inquisitive.
- Diversity – create, foster, and maintain a culturally diverse learning community.

- Excellence -- achieve our highest goals and become the best we can be.
- Integrity – maintain the highest respect, trust and ethical standards in all our interactions and activities.
- Leadership – educate and train physicians, researchers, and other health care professionals to become leaders in their fields at a regional, state and national level.
- Learning – develop strategies for life-long, self-directed learning, sharing of knowledge, and translating new concepts to practice.
- Responsibility - exhibit a strong sense of duty, stewardship and accountability to each other and to our varied constituencies.

Partners and Resources

The Dell Medical School is supported by an extraordinary group of partner organizations all committed to the development, growth, and success of a world-class institution. These partners have invested unprecedented resources and expertise towards the launch of the school:

The University of Texas System operates nine academic UT campuses and six health

science centers. The Board of Regents has approved the creation of the Dell Medical School, clearing the way for a decision by the Higher Education Coordinating Board on whether The University of Texas at Austin may offer an MD degree. The Board of Regents has pledged funds for the construction of the Dell Medical School -- at least $25 million in continuing support and an additional $5 million annually for eight years -- for faculty recruitment and support.

Construction of a new University Medical Center Brackenridge is the job of **Seton Healthcare Family**. It will be a teaching hospital for Dell Medical School students, while also providing residencies to graduate and postgraduate medical education. Seton expects to commit $250 million to the hospital.

Seton operates more than 90 clinical locations including five major medical centers, two community hospitals, three rural hospitals, an inpatient mental health hospital, three primary care clinics for uninsured people and several strategically located health facilities. The system offers the region's only Level I trauma centers for adult and pediatric patients. Its insurance division works with commercial insurance companies, community physicians and Medicaid and Medical Access programs for low-income persons, to assist in the management of the region's overall health.

Seton is home to The University of Texas Southwestern (UTSW) Medical Center's Austin medical residency programs, as well as the Seton/UTSW Clinical Research Institute.

The organization's role in education, research and spiritual programming furthers Seton's mission to improve the health of the communities it serves, with special concern for the poor and the vulnerable, as it prepares the region's next generation of clinicians. In Fiscal Year 2011, Seton provided almost $350 million in charity care.

Seton is a member of Ascension Health, the nation's largest not-for-profit health network.

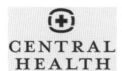

Created by Travis County voters in 2004, **Central Health** (the Travis County Healthcare District) provides health care coverage and funding through an extensive network of health care providers who offer access to care to low-income, uninsured residents of Travis County. Central Health is primarily funded by property tax revenues and lease payments from Seton Healthcare Family for University Medical Center Brackenridge (UMCB), which Central Health owns. Seton leases the hospital from Central Health and operates it on Central Health's behalf. Central Health and Seton also are partners in creating a new organization called the Community Care Collaborative. The Collaborative is designed to transform the delivery system to better coordinate services and funding for the benefit of those who most need access to health care in Travis County.

Central Health will leverage -- at a rate more than double -- the local investment in health care delivery with matching federal funds. As part of this plan, Central Health will purchase services from the Dell Medical School for the population it serves, resulting in $35 million in annual revenue to the medical school project. Travis County voters in November 2012 approved an increase in local property taxes from 7.89 cents per $100 valuation to 12.89 cents per $100 valuation, which will be used to support numerous innovative healthcare initiatives, including the Collaborative, Dell Medical School, the new teaching hospital and others.

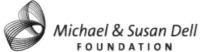

On Jan. 30, 2013 **the Michael & Susan Dell Foundation** announced a new $50 million commitment to establish the Dell Medical School at The University of Texas at Austin. Additionally, the Dell family foundation committed another $10 million to Austin and Travis County community health quality and access programs over the next 10 years. Since its inception in 1999, the foundation has invested nearly $1 billion in health and education programs around the globe, including $150 million during the past decade to promote family and childhood health in Central Texas.

Academic Philosophy

Students and faculty will be provided with the opportunity to conduct in-depth research in basic and translational sciences and medicine. They will test theories in the natural sciences, engineering and technology, business management and social sciences in clinics and state-of-the-art laboratories. The Dell Medical School will create opportunities for synergy among UT's existing schools and colleges of nursing, social work, pharmacy, natural sciences, engineering, education, liberal arts, public policy, and business. It will leverage research in areas as diverse as medical ethics and business systems to solve one of the most pressing issues facing America: how to create better health in the communities we serve.

From research bench to the patient clinic to bedside, it will be a fertile, inspirational academic environment for the intellectually curious student and for faculty members dedicated to discovery. This approach — interprofessional and transdisciplinary education — will train doctors who will pursue medicine with broad scientific and academic backgrounds, who love innovation and respect the contributions of all health care providers.

Research

The Dell Medical School will draw on the university's existing research strengths, including cell and molecular biology, neuroscience, biomedical engineering, chemistry, public health, sociology, psychology, health care delivery systems and health care policy. The school will also be integrated with the university's well-regarded programs in nursing, pharmacy and social work to prepare physicians for the health care system of the future and work collaboratively with a growing biotechnology industry in Central Texas. The result will be innovations that improve the way people receive health care. The research portfolio will balance basic, clinical and community research.

Facilities

An education/administration building and a research building are planned and will be funded through the UT System Board of Regents. The buildings will be located near the current site of University Medical Center Brackenridge and the university's School of Nursing. On May 9, the University of Texas Board of Regents approved a $334 million request for these facilities.

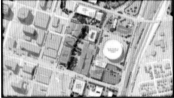

Seton has committed at least $250 million – a portion of which will come from fundraising --- to build a new teaching hospital to replace the aging University Medical Center Brackenridge. The hospital will serve as the medical school's primary clinical in-patient teaching facility and enhance services to residents of Central Texas. It will also upgrade the only Level I adult trauma center for a populous and growing 11-county area.

A team that includes the UT System, The University of Texas at Austin, Seton Healthcare Family and Central Health has been developing a master site plan for the placement of the school, the new teaching hospital, clinics and a medical office building. The area being studied is beyond the southeast corner of the university's campus, generally south of Martin Luther King Jr. Boulevard, west of Interstate 35 and east of Trinity Street, including the current site of University Medical Center at Brackenridge. The goal of the effort is to accommodate current needs while allowing for growth. The master plan also is being coordinated with the State of Texas, which is working on a master plan for state property in the adjacent Capitol area. Among the many planning dimensions are transportation, utilities, flooding and environmental concerns and general urban design.

Governance

To guide the early stages of building the Dell Medical School, a steering committee has been established, led by Dr. Sue Cox, interim senior associate dean, and Dr. Robert O. Messing, vice provost for biomedical sciences. The committee represents schools and colleges within The University of Texas at Austin as well as Seton Healthcare Family, Central Health and UT Southwestern Medical School. Its advisers include representatives of the University of Texas System and key UT Austin administrators.

Upon appointment, the Inaugural Dean will report directly to the Provost of The University of Texas at Austin but will also hold the title of Vice President, and as such will be considered part of the President's senior leadership team.

Accreditation

Earlier this year, the University of Texas System Regents gave preliminary approval to ask the Texas Higher Education Coordinating Board to authorize a Doctor of Medicine degree at the new medical school. The Dell Medical School must be accredited by the Liaison Committee on Medical Education (LCME) to be eligible for many federal grants, and students must study at an accredited school to qualify to take the U.S. Medical Licensing Examination. The LCME also requires that the sponsoring institution receive regional accreditation from the appropriate body. For Texas, that is the Southern Association of Colleges and Schools Commission on Colleges (SACS COC), and UT Austin is accredited as a Level VI school, offering 4 or more Doctoral Degrees.

Work is currently underway by the Steering Committee to prepare an outline that identifies the curriculum that the Dell Medical School will teach, and the target date to produce this in draft form is September 1, 2014. The target date to submit the LCME application is December, 2014 with the hope for preliminary accreditation in June, 2015.

The Role of the Dean of the Dell Medical School

The Inaugural Dean of the Dell Medical School ("the Dean") is the chief architect, executive and intellectual leader of the school. The Dean is responsible for building and ensuring the highest possible quality in medical, graduate, and post-graduate education and research. In addition, the Dean will be a key player in sustaining partnerships established with Seton Healthcare and Central Health that will assure the success of the new Dell Medical School and the growth of healthcare in the Austin region. The Dean is also responsible for matters relating to the design and effective administration of the Dell Medical School including academic programs, faculty, students, staff, facilities, resources, budgets, fundraising and relationships with the community and external stakeholders.

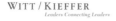

Opportunities and Expectations for Leadership

The key stakeholders leading the development and launch of the Dell Medical School have identified the following general goals and objectives:

- Build and lead an organization that will develop a strong reputation for excellence in education, for advancement in research and scholarly activities, for promotion of quality clinical training and service, and for a demonstrated commitment to community-based medical care.

- Recruit a first-class senior leadership team to whom the Dean can effectively delegate the key strategic and operational aspects of establishing a medical school.

- Build relationships and partnerships with Austin's leaders and serve as the "champion" who will inspire the community's enthusiasm and support for the Dell Medical School.

- In partnership with the academic leaders of The University of Texas at Austin, build a progressive, cutting edge curriculum that challenges and inspires students, and integrates many of the university's outstanding colleges, schools, centers, and programs in robust interdisciplinary initiatives.

- Build a culture of excellence in the Dell Medical School that incorporates fairness, integrity, respect, creativity, initiative and community service.

- Catalyze development of an innovation economy centered around biotechnology in Austin and Central Texas.

The following are specific leadership priorities that the Inaugural Dean will want to pay particular attention to in the earlier stages of his/her leadership tenure:

1. **Achieving successful accreditation** – Even with ample resources and partners in place, a new medical school cannot open without gaining LCME accreditation through a peer-review process designed to attest to the educational quality of new programs. The incoming Dean must immediately insure that accreditation plans are properly structured and on an appropriate time track for review and approval so that the first class can be recruited in the Fall of 2015.

2. **Defining clinical education partnerships** – The Seton Healthcare Family has sponsored extensive medical residency programs for years and has drawn on the engagement of many of the Travis County Medical Society's 3,200 physicians. Currently, Seton funds over 230 UT Southwestern residents in 16 residency and fellowship programs, 144 full-time faculty members, and 180 volunteer faculty members. In addition there are a total of 100 3rd and 4th year UTMB students on clinical rotations in Austin. Residents rotate at other clinical sites including community clinics, private doctor's office, and within St. David's Healthcare Partnership (Austin's second largest system). The Dean will need to fully appreciate the newly-defined roles, relationships and operating/financial arrangements of these partners.

3. **Building robust interdisciplinary opportunities** – The establishment of a new medical school within a world-class teaching and research university presents an enormous potential for developing powerful interdisciplinary and interprofessional programs that will extend the value of the medical school to all corners of the university. Appendix B offers a starting view of the many opportunities for collaboration. The Inaugural Dean should focus on learning about these different schools and their programs and building relationships with their leaders with an eye to quickly leveraging their collective strengths with the medical school.

4. **Finalize working agreements with key partners** – The agreements in principle that were developed prior to the Proposition 1 tax election will be replaced by detailed working agreements that include Seton Healthcare Family, Central Health (the Travis County health care district) and the university. These agreements will cover the assets to be constructed for the Dell Medical School effort and ongoing funding of medical school education, residency training and the provision of medical services. It will be essential that the Dean not only finalize formal agreements, but through this process ensure that all parties are aligned towards common goals. This will allow the Dell Medical School to serve as a "bridge" that connects its partners inside and outside of the university.

5. **Managing stakeholder expectations** – An enormous amount of excitement has been generated by this initiative, and a great deal of attention is centered on the establishment of the medical school by constituents in the university, the hospital community, the physician community, public/political leaders, taxpayers, the business sector, and the media. While all are aligned on the primary goal of building a world-class medical school, each constituency has a keen interest in the value that the medical school will add to their particular needs.

   For example, while The University of Texas at Austin's academic leaders are particularly focused on a school that will excel in teaching and research, the external communities are expecting their investments to yield a significant return in expanded access to high quality clinical care and that the school will serve as an economic development engine for the Austin region. These are not mutually exclusive aspirations and will be pursued in parallel. The Inaugural Dean will need to first understand and appreciate these expectations, and then ensure that the school and its programs ideally balance all of these in a way that continues the support and respect of these many and diverse stakeholders.

Personal Qualifications and Personal Qualities

The Inaugural Dean of the Dell Medical will be a strategic leader who is fully capable of managing a substantial, complex, evolving organization. Ideally, the Search Committee is seeking candidates who come from an academic medicine setting (i.e. medical school dean, associate/assistant dean, or department chair) whose style and leadership characteristics can be described as progressive, creative and innovative.

More specifically, the ideal candidate will possess or have demonstrated the vast majority of the following attributes:

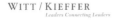

Education

- M.D., M.D./PhD. or equivalent degree is required;

- Board Certification in the candidate's specialty/discipline is required.

Preferred Experience

- Significant achievement in clinical, education and research pursuits; a personal record of accomplishment in collaborative research, a keen appreciation for interdisciplinary collaboration; and a personal commitment to human and population health research;

- Progressive and broad administrative leadership experience within an academic institution;

- A demonstrated history of innovative leadership, and conversant in current efforts to transform medical education using innovative curricula, technologies, and teaching/learning methodologies;

- Exceptional recruiting talents – can bring a vast personal network of relationships and choose talent in a way that extends leadership into the organization;

- Management experience in the "business" of medical schools: finances, research, accreditation, the challenges and operation of the clinical enterprise; strong fiscal skills and proven experience with budgets and grants management;

- Successful development or expansion of an organization or program; an acknowledged reputation in the building of exemplary clinical and research programs;

- Familiarity and understanding of entrepreneurship and technology commercialization in an academic medical setting;

- Appreciation for project management techniques and tools;

- Direct experience in serving in a high-profile role external to an institution – interacting regularly and effectively with political, community, private sector leaders and the media;

- Proven track record of cultivating the interest and involvement of both current and potential donors, resulting in the closing of major and principal gifts.

Preferred Leadership Qualifications and Personal Qualities

- Exceptional interpersonal and communication skills; a record of promoting collaboration and cultivating strong external relationships; and is a consensus and relationship builder "of the first order;"

- Artful and apt negotiation skills – applied towards the goal of forging "win-win" compromises;

- Ability to communicate an inspiring long-term vision for the future and be an articulate and engaging spokesperson for the school;

- History of bringing different organizations and individuals together to address common goals, a "leader among leaders;"

- Ability to project a genuine passion for an organization's mission and objectives;

- A collegial, consultative and diplomatic management style that respects and facilitates interdisciplinary cooperation;

- Ability to be strong, disciplined, decisive, to take calculated risks and to build organizations;

- Analytical skills and conceptual thinking that identifies opportunities and catalyzes action;

- Level of comfort in hands-on engagement in key areas, but with a sense of when and how to effectively delegate to others;

- Patient and able to thrive in a setting of ambiguity and change;

- High level of energy, enthusiasm, humor and optimism;

- Approachable and compassionate;

- Self-confident with political acumen and personal humility;

- Unquestioned personal integrity.

Austin, Texas

Austin is nestled among the rolling hills and lakes of Central Texas, the seat of state government, an educational Mecca with several area universities, home to a host of high tech companies including Dell Computers, Silicon Labs, Freescale, AMD, Samsung and many others related to the computer, semiconductor and internet industries. Austin is an entertainment center that includes the best of live music, the arts, and all the fun of the great outdoors.

Austin's weather has attracted many to this beautiful part of Texas; the blue skies and many sunny days are highly valued by its residents. Austin has its own professional symphony, ballet and opera companies, dozens of theaters, dance companies, vocal ensembles, and orchestras producing events year-round, as well as art museums, galleries, and beautiful sculpture gardens. With its many area universities and colleges and its award-winning public and private schools, Austin is a thriving educationally driven city.

The city's expanding health care system now rivals that of any major metropolitan area. Besides a number of major hospitals and one children's hospital, there are numerous out-patient clinics, emergency medical facilities, and all manner of awareness programs.

For much more information on Austin and its environs, please choose from the many websites available at http://www.utexas.edu/austin/.

Opportunity Summary

The Inaugural Dean of the Dell Medical School will be presented with the opportunity to achieve the following professional and personal goals:

➢ Serve on the senior leadership team of one of the most respected and renowned research universities in the United States.

➢ Play a signature role in the development and implementation of a new medical school whose success will enhance the quality and delivery of health care in all regions of the state and significantly enhance the medical education of new generations of physicians.

➢ Forge an historic cooperation among teachers, researchers and health care providers in state-of-the-art facilities in a common effort to produce the knowledge, management systems and skilled doctors who will improve the lives of millions of people, both locally and globally.

➢ Interact regularly with a diverse and collaborative group of senior leaders, including members of the Board of Regents, campus presidents, peer executives in the UT System office, and an outstanding staff.

➢ Reside in a region of Texas that is rich with history and intellectual tradition and offers a high quality of living in an affordable setting.

Procedure for Candidacy

Inquiries, nominations and applications are invited. Candidates should provide a *curriculum vitae*, a letter of application that addresses the responsibilities and requirements described in the Leadership Statement, and the names and contact information of five references. References will not be contacted without prior knowledge and approval of candidates. These materials should be sent electronically via e-mail to The University of Texas at Austin consultants, John K. Thornburgh, Brian Bloomfield and Michael M.E. Johns, M.D., at DellMedicalDean@wittkieffer.com.

Review of candidates for this position by the Dell Medical School Dean Search Committee will commence in September, 2013 and will continue until the position is filled, with the hope that the Inaugural Dean will assume office by early 2014. To make an inquiry please contact John K. Thornburgh at (412) 209-2666 or johnt@wittkieffer.com or Brian Bloomfield at (949) 797-3548 or brianb@wittkieffer.com. Materials that cannot be transmitted electronically may be sent to:

Inaugural Dean, Dell Medical School
The University of Texas at Austin
Attn: John K. Thornburgh
Witt/Kieffer
2015 Spring Road, Suite 510
Oak Brook, IL 60523

The University of Texas at Austin values diversity and is committed to equal opportunity for all persons regardless of age, color, disability, ethnicity, marital status, national origin, race, religion, sex, sexual orientation, veteran status or any other status protected by law.

Discover Thought Leadership at www.wittkieffer.com

The material presented in this position specification should be relied on for informational purposes only. This material has been copied, compiled, or quoted in part from The University of Texas at Austin documents and personal interviews and is believed to be reliable. While every effort has been made to ensure the accuracy of this information, the original source documents and factual situations govern.

Appendix A: Inaugural Dean Search Committee

The members of the search committee are:

Member	Affiliation
Robert O. Messing, Chair	Vice Provost for Biomedical Sciences
Reginald C. Baptiste	Capital Cardiothoracic Surgeons
Charles Barnett	Executive Chairman of the Board - Seton Healthcare Family, Austin, Texas
Da'marcus E. Baymon	Senior, UT Austin College of Natural Sciences
Susan Cox	UT Southwestern Regional Dean for Austin Programs
Lynn Crismon	Dean, UT Austin College of Pharmacy
Gregory L. Fenves	Dean, UT Austin Cockrell School of Engineering
J. Gregory Fitz	Executive Vice President for Academic Affairs and Provost, Dean of UT Southwestern Medical School
Francisco González-Scarano	Dean of the School of Medicine and Vice President for Medical Affairs at the UT Health Science Center at San Antonio
Andrea Gore	Professor, College of Pharmacy
Clarke Heidrick	Central Health Board of Managers
Linda Hicke	Dean, UT Austin College of Natural Sciences
Dan Johnston	Chair of Neurobiology Section, UT Austin College of Natural Sciences
Alan Lambowitz	Director of the Institute for Cellular and Molecular Biology, UT Austin
James O. Lindsey	Senior Vice President, Medical Affairs and Chief Medical Officer, Seton Healthcare Family
Russell Poldrack	Director, Imaging Research Center, UT Austin College of Liberal Arts

| Stephanie Tutak | Junior, UT Austin College of Natural Sciences |
| Mary Velasquez | Associate Dean for Research, UT Austin School of Social Work |

Appendix B: Potential Interdisciplinary Collaborations

Cockrell School of Engineering

Drug discovery and delivery
Biomaterials
Biomechanics
Gene therapy
Health information technologies and systems
Laser microsurgery
Nerve regeneration
Nanotechnology and microfluidics in medical systems
Protein drugs and diagnostics
Regenerative medicine and tissue engineering
Cardiovascular modeling
Computer aided cancer detection

College of Communication

Communication sciences and disorders
Health promotion and communication
Media coverage of health care, science
Patient education and counseling
Online patient support, e-visit programs

College of Education

Cardiovascular health
Exercise science
Muscle regeneration
Motor control
Spinal cord injury

College of Liberal Arts

Biomedical ethics
Cognitive neuroscience
Cultural influences on health care delivery
Global health and social medicine
Health policy
Human population genetics
Human and primate evolution
Perceptual systems
Population-level health disparities
Psychotherapy of mental disorders

College of Natural Sciences

Addiction
Aging
Birth defects and developmental biology
Cancer biology
Health information systems
Immunology
Infectious disease
Learning and memory
Neurodegenerative disease and Down's syndrome
Neurogenesis
Obesity and nutrition
Pain

College of Pharmacy

Addiction
Cancer biology
Drug design, delivery and metabolism
Endocrine disorders
Environmental toxicology
Health outcomes research
Infectious disease
Pain
Vaccine development and delivery

LBJ School of Public Affairs

Health care reform and innovation
Evaluation of health care practices and interventions
Economic and social outcomes of health care policy
Social policy and health

McCombs School of Business

Computer simulation for improved healthcare delivery
Improving use of electronic health records, accounting and financial metrics
Minority health, health care and health disparities
Organizational practices for better outcomes in healthcare organizations
Patient-centered medical care
Process analysis, scheduling and quality improvement
Structuring relationships of healthcare teams

School of Information

Health informatics

School of Law

Health law
Health policy
Medical ethics
Regulation and public policy
Science, technology and the law

School of Nursing

Adolescent health
Behavioral health interventions
Gerontology
Community-based interventions
Self-management of chronic illness

School of Social Work

Addiction
Behavioral health
Cancer care
Mental health

Institutes, Centers, and Graduate Programs

Center for Learning and Memory
Center for Advancement of Research and Education in Infectious Diseases
Center for Nano- and Molecular Science
Dell Pediatric Research Institute
Drug Dynamics Institute
Health behavior and research Training Institute
Institute for Computational Engineering and Sciences
Institute for Cellular and Molecular Biology
Institute for Neuroscience
Texas Advanced Computing Center
Texas Institute for Drug and Diagnostic Development
Texas Institute for Excellence in Mental Health
Waggoner Center for Alcohol and Addiction Research

Appendix C: Proposed Organization Chart

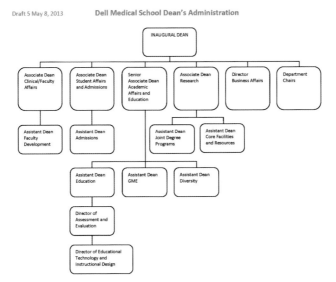

WITT / KIEFFER
Leaders Connecting Leaders

Witt/Kieffer is the preeminent executive search firm that identifies outstanding leadership solutions for organizations committed to improving the quality of life. The firm's values are infused with a passion for excellence, personalized service and integrity.

CHRONOLOGY

1881	Statewide Referendum on Location of Medical School
1884	Brackenridge Hospital Established
1890	UTMB—Old Red Built, 1891 Faculty Established
1910	Flexner Report
1931	First Rotating Intern, Brackenridge
1950	UTMB, Students in Austin
1958	Mayor's Committee on Austin Medical School
1959	UT South Texas Medical School—House Bill 9
1968	UT South Texas School Dedicated
1972	Central Texas Medical Foundation Established by TCMS
1980–1990	Brackenridge OB/GYN Residency Affiliated with UT Houston
1993	Formal Student Rotations from UTMB
1995	Seton Takes over Brackenridge
1996	Brackenridge Residency affiliated with UTMB
2003	CTI Research and Education in Medicine and Biotechnology Founded (UTMB Campus in Austin)
	Krusee/Stick Push for School in North Austin
November 2003	Guckian Papers on UTMB (Fifteen Acres at Mueller)
2004	Shine Memo to Regents on Austin Academic Health Center

2004 (*continued*)	Rumors of UTMB Moving to Austin
	Austin American-Statesman Oppel Editorial on Medical School
August 11, 2004	Shine Presentation to Regents on Academic Health Center
December 6, 2004	MD/PhD Program UTMB/UT Austin
Fall 2005	Dell Discussions
October 14, 2005	Presentation to Dells on Dell Medical School
November 2005	Dells' Interest in DPRI
	UTMB/Seton Thirty-Year Agreement on Residencies
January 12, 2006	Shine Presentation to Regents on Austin Academic Health Center
May 10, 2006	DPRI Naming Approved by Regents
July 14, 2006	Sam Shoemaker Appointed Dean of UTMB Regional Programs
August 22–23, 2007	PUF/STARs/AUF for DPRI
November 8–9, 2007	AUF/$25 Million to Austin for DPRI Faculty
2007	Perryman Report on Economic Benefits
2007–2008	Plan for Medical School Evolves
2008	Texas A&M Health Programs in Round Rock
	Economic Downturn Stops Development
December 2009	Seton/UTSW Agreement
October 28, 2010	DPRI Opens
February 2011	Amy Shaw Thomas, Kenneth Shine, Charles Barnett, Greg Hartman—Community Action Approach to Senator Kirk Watson
September 20, 2011	Watson's 10 Goals in 10 Years
May 2–3, 2012	Chancellor Recommends Medical School in Austin and South Texas with Funding for Austin
November 2, 2012	Huffines Op-Ed on Central Health Proposition 1
November 6, 2012	Central Health Proposition 1 passes
July 10, 2014	Agreement of UT Austin and Central Health Approved by Board of Regents
August 2014	Founding Dean Arrives Permanently
October 2014	First Hospital District Payment to UT Seton
May 2017	Dell Seton Medical Center at the University of Texas opens

NOTES

INTRODUCTION

1. Abraham Flexner, *Medical Education in the United States and Canada: A Report to the Carnegie Foundation for the Advancement of Teaching* (New York: The Carnegie Foundation for the Advancement of Teaching, 1910).

CHAPTER 1

1. Now the University of Texas at Austin.

2. Abraham Flexner, *Medical Education in the United States and Canada: A Report to the Carnegie Foundation for the Advancement of Teaching* (New York: The Carnegie Foundation for the Advancement of Teaching, 1910).

3. Flexner, *Medical Education*, 812.

4. Flexner, *Medical Education*, 812.

5. William Rothstein, *American Medical Schools and the Practice of Medicine: A History* (New York: Oxford University Press, 1987).

6. Rothstein, *American Medical Schools*, 150.

7. Rothstein, *American Medical Schools*, 150.

8. Rothstein, *American Medical Schools*, 150.

9. Flexner, *Medical Education*, 310–11.

10. *The University of Texas Medical Branch at Galveston: A Seventy-Five Year History by the Faculty and Staff* (Austin: The University of Texas Press, 1967).

11. UTMB, *A Seventy-Five Year History*, 10–11.

12. UTMB, *A Seventy-Five Year History*, 12.

13. UTMB, *A Seventy-Five Year History*, 12–15.

14. *Handbook of Texas*, Texas State Historical Association, "Ashbel Smith (1805–1886)," https://www.tshaonline.org/handbook/entries/smith-ashbel.

15. UTMB, *A Seventy-Five Year History*, 15.

16. UTMB, *A Seventy-Five Year History*, 16.

17. UTMB, *A Seventy-Five Year History*, 18.

18. UTMB, *A Seventy-Five Year History*, 18.

19. UTMB, *A Seventy-Five Year History*, 3.

20. James E. Thompson, "Medical College Faces Brightest Outlook in History" (speech), University of Texas, May 30, 1925, Austin, TX, 34th commencement of Medical Department.

21. "A Medical Wilderness: 1890 to 1939," *Southwestern Medical Perspectives* (Spring 2014): 5, https://swmedical.org/southwestern-medical-perspectives-spring-2014/.

22. "Building Momentum: 1955 to 1979," *Southwestern Medical Perspectives*, 45.

23. Will C. Sansom, *The Crown Jewel: The Story of the First 50 Years of the University of Texas Health Science Center at San Antonio* (Houston: UT Health Science, 2009), 9.

24. Sansom, *The Crown Jewel*, 9.

25. Sansom, *The Crown Jewel*, 9.

26. Sansom, *The Crown Jewel*, 19.

27. Sansom, *The Crown Jewel*, 12.

28. Sansom, *The Crown Jewel*, 11.

CHAPTER 2

1. "Regents Hear Medical Group: Board to Think over Medical School Policy," *Austin American-Statesman*, October 26, 1941.

2. "Medical School Controversy Is Simmering," *Austin American-Statesman*, March 2, 1942.

3. "Leake Defends Location of Medical School," *Austin American-Statesman*, December 9, 1944.

4. "Regents Hear Medical Group," *Austin American-Statesman*.

5. "Austin Becoming Medical Capital," *Austin American-Statesman*, October 17, 1954.

6. Al Williams, "Austin Presents New Case for Medical Branch," *Austin American-Statesman*, May 18, 1958.

7. "Medical Science School in Austin, 'Crash' Plea," editorial, *Austin American-Statesman*, July 2, 1961.

8. "Medical Science School."

9. "Medical Science School."

10. Chris Whitecraft, "Medical School 'Not for Austin,'" *Austin American-Statesman*, March 18, 1967.

11. "Seton Infirmary (600 W 26th St.)—1922," Reddit, accessed April 27, 2021, https://www.reddit.com/r/Austin/comments/acud3v/seton_infirmary_600 _w_26th_st_1922/.

CHAPTER 3

1. Frank Denius, personal communication, September 16, 2014.

2. "Medical Education Institute Created," *Austin Business Journal*, September 17, 2003.

3. Larry R. Faulkner, email message to James Guckian, April 8, 2002.

4. Faulkner, email message.

5. Faulkner, email message.

6. Faulkner, email message.

7. Faulkner, email message.

8. Faulkner, email message.

9. Faulkner, email message.

10. Austin Chamber of Commerce, *Opportunity Austin 2003*, February 2003.

11. Austin Chamber of Commerce, *Opportunity Austin 2003*.

12. Opportunity Austin, *The Economic Impact of the Primary Medical Sector on Austin's Economy*, August 2006.

13. Opportunity Austin, *The Economic Impact*.

14. Opportunity Austin, *The Economic Impact*.

15. Opportunity Austin, *The Economic Impact*.

16. "Medical Education Institute Created," *Austin Business Journal*.

17. The Perryman Group, *The Impact of Developing a Major Medical School at the University of Texas at Austin on the Regional and State Business Activity* (Austin, TX: Austin Chamber of Commerce, April 2007).

18. Perryman Group, *Impact*.

19. Perryman Group, *Impact*.

20. Perryman Group, *Impact*.

21. Perryman Group, *Impact*.

22. Perryman Group, *Impact*. Perryman noted, "Only two Texas medical schools made their [*U.S. News & World Report*] list of the top 50 research medical schools in the country for 2008." One reason for this relatively poor showing is that, in general, Texas medical schools are not located in close proximity to major universities and are unable to benefit from the affiliation.

23. Perryman Group, *Impact*.

24. Central Health, *Travis County Healthcare District Strategic Plan*, January 25, 2007.

25. Texas Perspectives, Inc., *Academic Medicine in Austin: Economic Implications*, fall 2011.

26. TXP, *Academic Medicine in Austin*.

27. TXP, *Academic Medicine in Austin*.

28. TXP, *Academic Medicine in Austin*.

29. TXP, *Academic Medicine in Austin*.

CHAPTER 4

1. Valerie M. Parisi to community, memorandum, July 14, 2006.

2. Parisi, memorandum.

3. Mary Ann Roser, "Uphill Fight for a Medical School," *Austin American-Statesman*, November 10, 2003.

4. Roser, "Uphill Fight."

5. Kenneth Shine, "Proposed Austin Academic Health Center" (presentation to Board of Regents, University of Texas System, Austin, TX, August 11, 2004).

6. Shine, "Austin Academic Health Center."

7. Jim Walker, email message to Kenneth Shine and others, January 24, 2006.

8. Heber Taylor, "An Opportunity for a Homegrown Institution," *Galveston Daily News*, July 24, 2005.

9. Taylor, "An Opportunity."

10. Taylor, "An Opportunity."

11. Taylor, "An Opportunity."

12. John Egan, "Seton Prepares to Unveil Deal with UTMB to Educate Medical Students," Capital Gains, *Austin Business Journal*, November 18–24, 2005.

13. Mary Ann Rankin, email message to Ben Streetman and others, January 16, 2006.

14. An academic health center is defined as the combination of medical education, medical research, and medical care, usually involving a medical school, a teaching hospital, and related facilities.

CHAPTER 5

1. William T. Solomon, letter to H. Scott Caven Jr., James Huffines, and Kenneth I. Shine, April 29, 2008.

2. Solomon, letter, April 29, 2008.

3. Solomon, letter, April 29, 2008.

4. Solomon, letter, April 29, 2008.

5. Kenneth I. Shine, letter to William T. Solomon, December 23, 2009.

CHAPTER 6

1. Ralph K. M. Haurwitz and Mary Ann Roser, "Watson Emphasizing Goal, Not Cost, When It Comes to Medical School," *Austin American-Statesman*, September 20, 2011.

2. Haurwitz and Roser, "Push for Medical School in Austin Gains Momentum," *Austin American-Statesman*, October 8, 2011.

3. Resolution of Central Health Board of Managers, August 15, 2012.

4. Katherine Haenschen, "St. David's Puts Corporate Profits over Community Health in Opposing Prop 1," *Burnt Orange Report*, October 24, 2012, https://thecontributor.com/st-davids-puts-corporate-profits-over-community-health-opposing-prop-1.

5. Rob Moshein, letter to the editor, *Austin American-Statesman*, October 14, 2012.

6. W. Gardner Selby, "Truth-O-Meter" feature, *Austin American-Statesman*, October 14, 2012.

7. Central Health, response to Prop 1 lawsuit, October 22, 2012.

8. Central Health, response to St. David's letter, October 24, 2012.

9. Central Health, response to St. David's letter, October 24, 2012.

10. Haenschen, "St. David's."

11. Haenschen, "St. David's."

12. Steve Leslie, email message to UT faculty, October 10, 2012.

13. Leslie, email message.

14. Ralph K. M. Haurwitz, "Watson Takes Glory, Risks on Medical School," *Austin American-Statesman*, October 24, 2012.

15. Haurwitz, "Watson Takes Glory."

16. Steve Leslie, email message to Amy Shaw Thomas, October 10, 2012.

17. Steve Leslie, email message to Janet Mountain, October 10, 2012.

18. Francisco Cigarroa, Chancellor's Message, November 1, 2012.

19. Cigarroa, Chancellor's Message.

CHAPTER 7

1. Haurwitz and Roser, "Critics Wary of Catholic Teaching Hospital for New UT Medical School," *Austin American-Statesman*, December 9, 2012; Haurwitz and Roser, "Catholic Rules at New Teaching Hospital Could Prompt Legal Action," *Austin American-Statesman*, July 22, 2013.

2. Kenneth Shine, email message to Jenny LaCoste-Caputo, comment for media, November 19, 2012.

BIBLIOGRAPHY

"A Medical Wilderness: 1890 to 1939," *Southwestern Medical Perspectives* (Spring 2014): 5, https://swmedical.org/southwestern-medical-perspectives spring -2014/.

"Austin Becoming Medical Capital." *Austin American-Statesman*, October 17, 1954.

Austin Chamber of Commerce, *Opportunity Austin 2003*, February 2003.

Central Health. Response to Prop 1 lawsuit, October 22, 2012.

Central Health. Response to St. David's letter, October 24, 2012.

Central Health. *Travis County Healthcare District Strategic Plan*, January 25, 2007.

Cigarroa, Francisco. Chancellor's Message, November 1, 2012.

Egan, John. "Seton Prepares to Unveil Deal with UTMB to Educate Medical Students." Capital Gains, *Austin Business Journal*, November 18–24, 2005.

Flexner, Abraham. *Medical Education in the United States and Canada: A Report to the Carnegie Foundation for the Advancement of Teaching*. New York: The Carnegie Foundation for the Advancement of Teaching, 1910.

Haenschen, Katherine. "St. David's Puts Corporate Profits over Community Health in Opposing Prop 1." *Burnt Orange Report*, October 24, 2012. https:// thecontributor.com/st-davids-puts-corporate-profits-over-community -health-opposing-prop-1.

Handbook of Texas. Texas State Historical Association. https://www.tshaonline .org.

Haurwitz, Ralph K. M., and Roser, Mary Ann. "Catholic Rules at New Teaching Hospital Could Prompt Legal Action." *Austin American-Statesman*, July 22, 2013.

Haurwitz, Ralph K. M., and Roser, Mary Ann. "Critics Wary of Catholic Teaching Hospital for New UT Medical School." *Austin American-Statesman*, December 9, 2012.

Haurwitz, Ralph K. M., and Roser, Mary Ann. "Push for Medical School in Austin Gains Momentum." *Austin American-Statesman*, October 8, 2011.

Haurwitz, Ralph K. M., and Roser, Mary Ann. "Watson Emphasizing Goal, Not Cost, When It Comes to Medical School." *Austin American-Statesman*, September 20, 2011.

"Leake Defends Location of Medical School." *Austin American-Statesman*, December 9, 1944.

"Medical Education Institute Created." *Austin Business Journal*, September 17, 2003.

"Medical School Controversy Is Simmering." *Austin American-Statesman*, March 2, 1942.

"Medical Science School in Austin, 'Crash' Plea." Editorial, *Austin American-Statesman*, July 2, 1961.

Moshein, Rob. Letter to the editor. *Austin American-Statesman*, October 14, 2012.

Opportunity Austin. *The Economic Impact of the Primary Medical Sector on Austin's Economy*, August 2006.

Perryman Group. *The Impact of Developing a Major Medical School at the University of Texas at Austin on the Regional and State Business Activity*. Austin, TX: Austin Chamber of Commerce, April 2007.

"Regents Hear Medical Group: Board to Think over Medical School Policy." *Austin American-Statesman*, October 26, 1941.

Resolution of Central Health Board of Managers, August 15, 2012.

Roser, Mary Ann. "Uphill Fight for a Medical School." *Austin American-Statesman*, November 10, 2003.

Rothstein, William G. *American Medical Schools and the Practice of Medicine: A History*. New York: Oxford University Press, 1987.

Sansom, Will C. *The Crown Jewel: The Story of the First 50 Years of the University of Texas Health Science Center at San Antonio*. Houston: UT Health Science, 2009.

Selby, W. Gardner. "Truth-O-Meter" feature. *Austin American-Statesman*, October 14, 2012.

"Seton Infirmary (600 W 26th St.)—1922." Reddit. Accessed April 27, 2021. https://www.reddit.com/r/Austin/comments/acud3v/seton_infirmary_600 _w_26th_st_1922/.

Shine, Kenneth I. "Proposed Austin Academic Health Center." Presentation to Board of Regents, University of Texas, Austin, TX, August 11, 2004.

The University of Texas Medical Branch at Galveston: A Seventy-Five Year History by the Faculty and Staff. Austin: The University of Texas Press, 1967.

Thompson, James E. "Medical College Faces Brightest Outlook in History." Speech. University of Texas, May 30, 1925, Austin, TX, 34th commencement of Medical Department. Transcript. https://texashistory.unt.edu/ark:/67531 /metapth821411/.

Weiskotten, Herman G. *Medical Education in the United States, 1934–1939.* Chicago: American Medical Association, 1940.

Williams, Al. "Austin Presents New Case for Medical Branch." *Austin American-Statesman,* May 18, 1958.

INDEX

Page numbers in italic indicate photographs.

instruction, 45; Shoemaker as dean, 72; and UTMB, 18, 75

Texas Education Code §74.201, 116, 206

Texas Health and Human Services Commission, 119

Texas Higher Education Coordinating Board, ix, 4, 116, 124, 206–7, 171

Texas Medical Association, 16, 21, 23, 29–30

Texas Medical Center (Houston), 4, 13, 21, 26

Texas medical schools, 1–2, 11–12; Baylor College of Medicine, 2, 9, 13–14, 20–21, 28, 104; early attempts in Austin, 29–32; Galveston, 16–17, 28; South Texas, 125; Texas Medical College and Hospital, 15; UT Southwestern (Dallas), 20–22; UTHSC-Houston, 25–26; UTHSC-San Antonio, 22–25; vote for location of (1881), 15–16. *See also* academic/medical school locations; Dell Medical School; teaching hospitals; UTMB

Texas Perspectives, Inc., 62–63, 66–67

Texas Pharmacy Congress medication error summit, 147–54

Texas State Journal of Medicine, 29

Texas System Board of Regents. *See* Board of Regents

Texas Tech University, 2, 9, 124

Theriault, Sean, 194

Thomas, Amy Shaw, viii, x–xi, x, 6, 41, 88, 104, 114, 128, 246; and AARO, 66; boards, committees, 143, 192, 198, 199; and CTI, 56; early discussion of Austin medical school, 38–40, 54, 72, 108, 111; and foundational affiliation agreements, 139; and Framework preparation, 115; and "hospital within a hospital" concerns, 35; outreach to commu-

nity leaders, 92, 116–18; and Proposition 1, 128; and residency issue, 103; and Stobo expansion efforts, 72; as Vice Chancellor, Counsel for Health Affairs, 141; and Watson, 126

Thompson, James E., 18

Thornburgh, John K., 224–44

Timmerman, Gayle, 194

Travis County: healthcare delivery model, 123–24; indigent care system, 65, 123; Medical Society, 32–33, 36–37, 119, 173; Prop 1 tax increase for, 120. *See also* Austin, Texas/City of Austin

Travis County Healthcare District. *See* Central Health

Troutman, Edwin G., 30

Turner, Jerry S., 56

Tutak, Stephanie, 223, 239

TXP (Texas Perspectives, Inc.), 62–63, 66–67

Tyler, Diane, 197

Ulman, Doug, 119, 199, 210

University of North Texas system, 9

University of Pennsylvania, 11–12

UT Austin, 88; DPRI operation given to, 93–94, 98, 100–102; and eminent domain, 81–82; and polarization among regents, 114–15; and UTMB, 30, 35, 38, 69, 75, 100, 103, 171–75

UT Austin medical school issues: affiliation, competition agreements, 139; "Anyone but the Yankees" syndrome, 58; and athletics programs, 104; budget concerns, 4–5, 86–87; communication and oversight, 20; CTI concerns regarding, 74, 77; debate over location, 4, 18–19, 109; early interest in, 28–33, 38, 100, 108–10; Galveston connection to, 1–2, 16; mobilizing community support, 44–45; motivations for, x; and